Auscultation Skills

Breath & Heart Sounds

Auscultation Skills

Breath & Heart Sounds

SPRINGHOUSE CORPORATION

Springhouse, Pennsylvania

Staff

Executive director
Matthew Cahill

Clinical director
Judith Schilling McCann, RN, MSN

Art director
John Hubbard

Managing editor
H. Nancy Holmes

Clinical project manager
Collette Bishop Hendler, RN, CCRN

Editors
Jane V. Cray, Vijay S. Kothare, Doris Weinstock

Copy editors
Cynthia C. Breuninger (manager), Deborah Arnold, Brenna H. Mayer, Pamela Wingrod

Designers
Arlene Putterman (associate art director), Lesley Weissman-Cook (designer), StellarVisions (project manager)

Cover illustration
Heidi Merscher

Book illustrations
The Turner Group

Typography
Diane Paluba (manager), Joyce Rossi Biletz, Valerie Molettiere

Manufacturing
Deborah Meiris (director), Patricia K. Dorshaw (manager), Otto Mezei (book production manager)

Editorial assistants
Beverly Lane, Marcia Mills, Liz Schaeffer

Indexer
Barbara Hodgson

Breath and heart sounds
Electronically generated by the Cardionics Respiration Sound Simulator and the Cardionics Heart Sound Simulator as per license from Cardionics.

Printed in the United States of America.

AUSCIL-D
02 01 00   10 9 8 7 6 5 4

Library of Congress Cataloging-in Publication Data

Auscultation skills: Breath & heart sounds.
       p. cm.
Includes bibliographical references and index.
1. Auscultation. I. Springhouse Corporation.
[DNLM: 1. Heart Auscultation — methods handbooks.
2. Heart Sounds — physiology handbooks.
3. Respiratory Sounds — physiology handbooks.
     WF 39A932 1998]
DC76.3.A97 1998
616.1'207544 — dc21
DNLM/DLC   98-11711
ISBN 0-87434-962-1   CIP

Contents

■

SECTION I:
Breath Sound Fundamentals

■

SECTION II:
Normal Breath Sounds

■

SECTION III:
Abnormal Breath Sounds

14 The third and fourth heart sounds 115

Pretest, Ventricular filling sounds, Third heart sound, Fourth heart sound, S_3 and S_4: Similarities and differences, Posttest

SECTION VII:
Abnormal Heart Sounds

15 Other diastolic and systolic sounds 126

Pretest, Opening snaps, Systolic ejection sounds, Posttest

16 Murmur fundamentals 134

Pretest, Turbulent blood flow, Characteristics, Posttest

17 Systolic murmurs 138

Pretest, Anatomy and physiology, Systolic ejection murmurs, Ventricular outflow obstruction murmurs, Systolic regurgitation murmurs, Ventricular septal defect murmur, Posttest

18 Diastolic murmurs 156

Pretest, Aortic regurgitation murmurs, Pulmonic regurgitation murmurs, Other diastolic murmurs, Posttest

19 Continuous murmurs 166

Pretest, Two causes, Cervical venous hum murmurs, Patent ductus arteriosus murmurs, Posttest

20 Other auscultatory sounds 170

Pretest, Prosthetic valve sounds and murmurs, Aortic prosthetic valves, Mitral prosthetic valves, Pericardial friction rubs, Mediastinal crunch, Posttest

Audiotape cues

Breath Sounds

The following breath sounds can be heard on the breath sounds audiotape that accompanies this book.

SIDE 1
  1. Tracheal and mainstem bronchi breath sounds
  2. Normal breath sounds heard over other chest wall areas
  3. Bronchovesicular breath sounds
  4. Bronchophony (normal)
  5. Egophony (normal)
  6. Whispered pectoriloquy (normal)
7, 8. Tracheal and mainstem bronchi breath sounds
  9. Normal breath sounds (midlung)
 10. Normal breath sounds (apex)
 11. Repeat #9
12, 13. Bronchial breath sounds (consolidation)
14, 15. Bronchial breath sounds (atelectasis)
16, 17. Bronchial breath sounds (fibrosis)
 18. Bronchophony (consolidation)
 19. Bronchophony (normal)
 20. Repeat #18
 21. Whispered pectoriloquy (atelectasis)
 22. Whispered pectoriloquy (normal)
 23. Repeat #21
 24. Egophony (tumor, pleural effusion)
 25. Egophony (normal)
 26. Repeat #24
 27. Diminished breath sounds (shallow breathing)
 28. Diminished breath sounds (diaphragmatic paralysis)
 29. Absent breath sounds (pneumothorax)
 30. Normal breath sounds
 31. Repeat #29
 32. Diminished breath sounds (pleural effusion)
 33. Normal breath sounds
 34. Repeat #32
35, 36. Diminished breath sounds (hyperinflated lungs)

37. Diminished breath sounds (obesity)
38. Diminished breath sounds (PEEP)

SIDE 2

39. Coarse crackles
40. Fine crackles
41. Wheezes
42. Low-pitched wheezes
43, 44. Late inspiratory crackles (atelectasis)
45, 46. Late inspiratory crackles (lobar pneumonia)
47, 48. Late inspiratory crackles (interstitial fibrosis)
49, 50. Late inspiratory crackles (left ventricular heart failure)
51, 52. Early inspiratory crackles (chronic bronchitis)
53, 54. Early to midinspiratory crackles (bronchiectasis)
55, 56. Pleural crackles
57, 58. Expiratory polyphonic wheezes
59, 60. Fixed monophonic wheezes
61, 62. Sequential inspiratory wheezes
63, 64. Random monophonic wheezes
65, 66. Stridor

Heart Sounds

The following heart sounds can be heard on the heart sounds audiotape that accompanies this book.

SIDE 1

1, 2. Normal S_1 and S_2 (base of heart)
3. S_1 (mitral area)
4. S_1 split so M_1 and T_1 can be heard better on expiration (tricuspid area)
5. Repeat of #3
6. Repeat of #4
7. Abnormal S_1 split
8, 9. S_2 (pulmonic area)
10, 11. S_2 split during inspiration and expiration
12. Increased intensity of P_2
13. Increased intensity of A_2
14. Diminished A_2
15. S_2 split during inspiration and expiration
16. Paradoxical S_2 split heard during expiration
17. Persistent S_2 split

18. Persistent S_2 split in pulmonary hypertension
19, 20. Wide, fixed S_2 split
21. Paradoxical S_2 split
22. Fused paradoxical S_2 split
23, 24. S_3 over mitral area (S_1, S_2, S_3)
25, 26. Abnormal S_3
27, 28. Pericardial knock
29, 30. Right-sided S_3
31, 32. S_4 (S_4, S_1, S_2)
33. Summation gallop
34. Right-sided S_4
35, 36. Opening snap of mitral valve
37, 38. Pulmonic ejection sound
39, 40. Aortic ejection sound
41, 42. Midsystolic click
43, 44. Innocent systolic ejection murmur
45, 46. Supravalvular pulmonic stenosis murmur

SIDE 2

47, 48. Pulmonic valvular stenosis murmur
49, 50. Subvalvular pulmonic stenosis murmur
51, 52. Supravalvular aortic stenosis murmur
53, 54. Aortic valvular stenosis murmur
55, 56. Subvalvular aortic stenosis murmur
57, 58. Tricuspid regurgitation murmur
59, 60. Holosystolic mitral regurgitation murmur
61, 62. Acute mitral regurgitation murmur
63. Mitral valve prolapse murmur with click
64. Mitral valve prolapse murmur
65, 66. Early diastolic aortic regurgitation murmur
67, 68. Austin Flint murmur
69, 70. Graham Steell murmur
71, 72. Normal pressure pulmonic valve murmur
73, 74. Mitral stenosis murmur (atrial fibrillation)
75. Mitral stenosis murmur (normal sinus rhythm)
76, 77. Tricuspid stenosis murmur
78, 79. Cervical venous hum murmur
80, 81. Patent ductus arteriosus murmur
82. Aortic prosthetic valve sound and murmur
83. Mitral prosthetic valve sound and murmur
84, 85. Pericardial friction rub
86, 87. Mediastinal crunch

Clinical consultants

Thomas A. Blackwell, MD
Assistant Professor of Medicine
University of Texas Medical Branch
Galveston

Virginia Butler, RN, BSN, MS
Creative Specialists, Inc.
Tulsa, Okla.

Jill M. Curry, RN, BSN, CCRN
Staff Nurse
Cardiac Care Unit
Hospital of the University of Pennsylvania
Philadelphia

Diane M. Czlonka, RN, MS, MA
Coordinator, Bioethics Program
Pulmonary Clinical Nurse Specialist
Detroit (Mich.) Medical Center—Sinai Hospital

Antonio G. deLeon, Jr., MD
Medical Director
St. John Cardiovascular Institute
St. John Medical Center
Tulsa, Okla.

Lyla Lindholm, RN, MN, CS
Pulmonary Clinical Nurse Specialist
St. Luke's Hospital
Kansas City, Mo.

Barbara C. Martin, RN, MS, CS
Professor of Nursing
University of Tulsa (Okla.)

Mary A. Stahl, RN, MSN, CS, CCRN
Cardiovascular Clinical Nurse Specialist
Saint Luke's Hospital
Kansas City, Mo.

Carol A. Stephenson, RN,C, EdD, CRNH
Associate Professor
Texas Christian University—Harris College of Nursing
Fort Worth

Foreword

In today's world of high-tech medicine, auscultation is quickly becoming a lost art. Advances in the field of chest radiography (such as computed tomography [CT] scanning and magnetic resonance imaging, angiography, and ultrasonography) have led many medical professionals to rely on these tests for diagnosis rather than auscultation and physical diagnosis. The typical response is, "Let's see what the chest X-ray or CT scan shows." This is a pity, as it contributes to distancing the health care professional from the patient.

Today, many health care professionals lack skill in auscultation and the stethoscope has become an ornament used mainly for blood pressure measurements. Invented in 1818, the stethoscope was originally used to identify the typical breath sounds heard in the diseases of the time: tuberculosis, pneumonia, bronchiectasis, emphysema, and lung cancer. With the resurgence of tuberculosis, the high incidence of heart failure and myocardial infarction, and the increasing incidence of lung cancer, the need for skillful auscultation is on the rise.

Skilled listening to your patient's lungs and heart permits early recognition of subtle changes in your patient's condition. This can, for example, give you time to forestall complications of heart failure. Auscultation may not only directly improve the relationship between you and your patient but also potentially decrease the cost of medical care by avoiding expensive — and possibly, with the help of auscultation expertise, unnecessary — tests.

Auscultation Skills: Breath and Heart Sounds and the accompanying audiotapes provide a practical tool to improve your ability to auscultate for these sounds and enhance your understanding of their physiology. By using this book together with the audiotapes and referring to them time and time again, you can review each breath and heart sound until you recognize it perfectly.

This invaluable book explains the physiology and pathophysiology of more than 40 different breath sounds and more than 50 different heart sounds. Illustrations highlight each system's anatomy as well as areas affected by, and auscultatory sites for, the sounds discussed.

The accompanying audiotapes provide electronically generated examples of nearly all the breath and heart sounds in the book. Breath sound examples begin with normal inspiration to make it easier for you to determine where the abnormality occurs in the respiratory cycle. Heart sounds start with S_1 to ease your recognition of abnormalities in the cardiac cycle.

The characteristics of breath and heart sounds are often very subtle and difficult to recognize. Perfecting the skill of auscultation requires not only a great deal of practice but also the opportunity to hear all of the sounds encountered in patient care.

We recommend that you first go through the book and tapes sequentially, and then go through again to review the sounds that you find difficult. A diamond (♦) appears in the text whenever you should turn on the tape. To ease your review of specific sounds, we've left a space in the text next to each auscultation cue. The first time you listen to the tape, set your tape player's counter to 000. Then, in the space we've provided, write the counter number for each breath or heart sound as you encounter it. Before you listen to the tape each time, be sure to return your tape counter to 000 to ensure an accurate match. Equipment varies, so if you periodically switch recorders, create a new set of numbers for each one.

Use the handy self-tests at the beginning and end of each chapter to check your knowledge of breath and heart sounds. You'll find detailed posttest answers at the back of the book.

Throughout the text, you'll find numerous auscultation tips and alerts. The auscultation tips advise you of sites and techniques to detect tricky sounds. The alerts warn you of life-threatening auscultation findings that demand an urgent response. For quick reference, we've compiled a glossary of commonly used terms and abbreviations and an easy-to-read chart of common disorders matched with specific abnormal sounds.

With all of this information at your fingertips, you'll be well on your way to perfecting your auscultation technique and interpretive skills. As we move into the 21st century, we need to combine technology with artful differential auscultation if we're to keep in touch with our patients and advance humanism in health care. *Auscultation Skills: Breath and Heart Sounds* is a great start.

Michael L. Lippmann, MD
Head, Pulmonary Division
Albert Einstein Medical Center
Philadelphia

Carol Twomey, RN, MSN, CRNP
Heart Transplant Nurse Coordinator
Allegheny-Hahnemann University Hospital
Philadelphia

SECTION I

Breath Sound
Fundamentals

1

The respiratory system and auscultation

▶❚ *PRETEST*

1. What is the primary function of the respiratory system?
2. Name two anatomic structures of the upper airway.
3. Name the anatomic structures of the lungs that are responsible for oxygen–carbon dioxide exchange.
4. What are the alveoli?
5. What are the roles of the airways' mucus layer and cilia?
6. What are the apex and base of the lung?
7. What is surfactant?
8. Name the two blood supplies in the lungs.
9. How is the lower airway innervated?
10. What are the pleurae?
11. What are the muscles of respiration?
12. Describe the process of normal breathing.
13. Are ventilation and blood flow equally distributed in the lungs?
14. What three chest wall surfaces are included in breath sound auscultation?
15. Is the diaphragm of a stethoscope ideally suited to transmit high-pitched or low-pitched sounds?
16. What is the auscultatory sequence?
17. What does contralateral comparison mean?
18. Does patient position affect breath sounds?

Anatomy and physiology

The respiratory system's primary function is the exchange of oxygen (O_2) and carbon dioxide (CO_2) between the alveoli and the pulmonary circulation.

During inspiration, air enters the upper airway and travels through the lower airways until it reaches the alve-

CO_2–O_2 exchange and airflow pattern during inspiration

Trachea

Bronchi

O_2 O_2

CO_2 CO_2

O_2 O_2

CO_2–O_2 exchange at alveolar-capillary membrane

oli. Each alveolus is surrounded by multiple capillaries. During systole, deoxygenated blood returning from the body's cells is pumped from the right ventricle through the arterial pulmonary circulation to the alveolar capillaries. CO_2 diffuses from the capillary blood across the alveolar capillary membrane and enters the alveolar air. Simultaneously, O_2 from the inspired atmospheric air in the alveolus crosses the alveolar capillary membrane and enters the pulmonary capillary blood.

During expiration, CO_2 is exhaled from the lungs. Oxygenated capillary blood travels to the heart's left side and is pumped from the ventricle into arterial circulation to the body's cells, where cellular respiration occurs. (See *CO_2–O_2 exchange and airflow pattern during expiration,* page 4.)

Upper airway

The upper airway consists of the nasal cavities and the pharynx. Air enters the body through the nostrils and passes through the nasal cavities. Large hairs located in the nostrils filter out foreign particles. The lateral walls of the nasal cavities curve, forming turbinates (conchae) that increase the mucosal surface area and produce turbulent airflow. (See *Location of turbinates and airflow pattern in nasal cavity,* page 4.) The lining of the nasal cavities con-

Location of nasal cavity and pharynx

1
2

1. Nasal cavity
2. Pharynx

CO_2–O_2 exchange and airflow pattern during expiration

Trachea

Bronchi

CO_2

CO_2

CO_2

CO_2

O_2

O_2

CO_2–O_2 exchange at alveolar-capillary membrane

Location of turbinates and airflow pattern in nasal cavity

1. Turbinates
2. Airflow

tains a dense capillary network and serous glands that warm and humidify the inspired air. Seromucous glands produce a sticky film over the lining that traps particles against it during airflow.

The *pharynx* is divided into three sections: the nasopharynx, the oropharynx, and the hypopharynx. The nasopharynx begins at the posterior openings of the nasal cavities and extends to the soft palate; the oropharynx, the middle section, is the common passageway for food and air; and the hypopharynx, the lower third of the pharynx, extends from the roof of the tongue to the glottic area.

Lower airway

The lower airway is called the *tracheobronchial tree*. It begins at the larynx and ends at the distal bronchioles, which open into the alveoli.

The *larynx*, which contains the epiglottis and vocal cords, has a role in ventilation and phonation and helps protect the lower airway from aspiration.

The *trachea* in a 154-lb (70-kg) adult male is approximately ¾″ to 1″ (2 to 2.5 cm) in diameter and 2¾″ (7 cm) long. (See *Location of trachea, right and left mainstem bronchi, and segmental and lobar bronchi,* page 6.) Anteriorly, the trachea begins just below the larynx and is located within the thoracic cavity, beneath the upper two-thirds of the sternum. Posteriorly, it begins at the level of the sixth cervical or first thoracic vertebra and extends to approximately the fifth thoracic vertebra.

The trachea divides into a right and left mainstem bronchus. The left mainstem bronchus leaves the trachea at a sharper angle than the right mainstem bronchus and passes under the aortic arch before entering the lung. The *mainstem bronchi* enter the lungs at the hila, where the lung tissue attaches to the mediastinum. The bronchi course downward and immediately divide into lobar bronchi, which subdivide into segmental bronchi.

The airways continue to systematically branch, narrow, shorten, and increase in number toward the lung periphery. They divide approximately 25 times before ultimately opening into the terminal, or respiratory, bronchioles.

The *terminal bronchioles,* which have a few alveoli budding from their walls, branch into alveolar ducts that are completely lined with alveoli. (See *Location of terminal bronchiole, alveolar duct, and alveoli,* page 7.) These airways and their alveoli form the respiratory lobules of the lungs. The terminal bronchioles account for the last six or seven airway divisions. The distance from the terminal bronchiole to the most distal alveolus is only about 5 mm; however, the majority of the lung surface area available for gas exchange is contained in these spaces.

The airways between the nose and the terminal bronchioles are called the *conducting airways.* Approximately 150 cc of inspired air remains in the conducting airways during each breath. This air, called *anatomic dead space,* is not involved in gas exchange.

The large airways below the glottis contain cartilage, smooth muscle, elastic fibers, connective tissue, and mucous glands. The trachea and mainstem bronchi are supported by anterior U-shaped cartilage. The cartilage that opens posteriorly is connected by a band of smooth muscle and fibroelastic tissue. Approximately 30% of the wall thickness in the mainstem and lobar bronchi is cartilage. This cartilage becomes irregular and platelike and eventually disappears in the smaller airways, which consist solely of smooth muscle and elastic fibers.

The mucous and bronchial glands located in the bronchial walls secrete a serous mucus blanket onto the inside airway walls. This secreted mucus forms a thin, sticky layer that lies on top of ciliated columnar epithe-

Location of nasopharynx, oropharynx, and hypopharynx

1. Nasopharynx
2. Oropharynx
3. Hypopharynx

Location of larynx, epiglottis, and vocal cords

1. Epiglottis
2. Vocal cords
3. Larynx

Location of trachea, right and left mainstem bronchi, and segmental and lobar bronchi

lial cells, which line nearly all of the respiratory tract between the larynx and the terminal bronchioles. The mucus layer traps foreign particles in the inspired air before they can enter the lungs. Cilia move in a wavelike motion, propelling the sticky mucus layer toward the pharynx where it can be coughed out or swallowed. Together, the mucus layer and cilia protect the lungs, acting as a major defense mechanism against inhaled particles.

Each lung is divided into lobes. The right lung has three lobes: the upper, middle, and lower. The left lung has only an upper and a lower lobe. The lung's apex (superior aspect) is located near the clavicle, and its base (inferior aspect) is located near the diaphragm. (See *Lung lobes*, page 8.)

Alveoli

The terminal bronchioles divide into 2 to 5 alveolar ducts, each of which consists of 10 to 16 alveoli. Alveoli contain three cell types. Type I, the largest, is the lining cell and accounts for 95% of the alveolar surface area. The type II cell produces surfactant, a mixture of phospholipids. The macrophage, the third cell type, acts as a phagocytic defense mechanism against infection.

The adult respiratory system contains approximately 300 million alveoli. In a healthy adult, the surface area of the alveolar-capillary membrane available for O_2–CO_2 ex-

Location of terminal bronchiole, alveolar duct, and alveoli

Terminal bronchiole

Alveolar duct

Alveoli

change is approximately 70 to 85 m², about the size of a tennis court.

The alveolar surface is covered by a fluid layer containing surfactant. Surfactant mixes with pulmonary fluids and maintains alveolar stability by lowering the alveolar surface tension, thus preventing the air-filled alveoli from collapsing at low volumes from the weight of capillary blood.

Lower airway innervation

Two neural pathways, the parasympathetic and sympathetic nervous systems, innervate the tracheobronchial tree. The relative balance of the two neural pathways and their effect on the smooth muscle, which lines the tracheobronchial tree, results in bronchial smooth muscle tone.

The parasympathetic nervous system in the larynx, trachea, and bronchi includes vagal nerve fibers and irritant receptors mediated by the neurotransmitter acetylcholine. Parasympathetic stimulation precipitates bronchoconstriction, coughing, and mucus discharge from the bronchial glands. Irritant receptors within the airways are believed to be responsible for increasing ventilation and precipitating coughing.

Sympathetic innervation of the lower airways usually arises from the thoracic nerves T1 through T5 and is mediated by the postganglionic hormone transmitter norepinephrine. Sympathetic stimulation of adrenergic beta$_2$-

Lung lobes

Apex

Right upper lobe

Right middle lobe

Right lower lobe

Left upper lobe

Left lower lobe

Diaphragm

Base

receptors throughout the lower airways facilitates smooth muscle relaxation, resulting in bronchodilation.

Secretory mast cells on the surface of the large airways also may be stimulated or affected by drugs, hormones, antigens, and other messenger cells to precipitate or control bronchoconstriction.

Pulmonary and bronchial circulation

Two blood supplies, the pulmonary and bronchial circulations, facilitate gas exchange and nourish the airways and other lung tissues.

The *pulmonary circulation* begins as the pulmonary artery leaves the right ventricle. The pulmonary artery divides into segmental arteries, which subdivide, ending in the pulmonary capillary bed surrounding the alveoli. The capillaries then join to form venules, which converge to form veins, then pulmonary veins. The pulmonary veins end in the left atrium.

The *bronchial circulation* usually originates in the aorta and branches along the bronchi to provide oxygen and nutrients to the lung tissue and to clear metabolic wastes from the airways and other lung tissues. Oxygenated blood is pumped from the aorta to the tracheobronchial tree and travels through arterioles along the airways. Deoxygenat-

Posterior view of thorax

Vertebral column

Ribs

ed blood from the bronchial circulation is returned to the left atrium, accounting for the normal 2% to 3% right-to-left shunt.

Pleurae

The chest wall's inner surface and the lungs' outer surfaces are joined by thin, membranous tissues called the *pleurae*. The parietal pleura covers the chest wall's inner surface, and the visceral pleura covers the lungs' outer surfaces. A small amount of fluid exists between the two layers. The pleurae separate into the right and left pleural cavities, which contain the lungs. During expansion and contraction of the chest wall and lungs, the pleurae glide smoothly and silently over each other.

The mechanics of breathing

The *thorax* is the bony structure that protects the vital organs (the heart and lungs) and permits chest expansion during inspiration. Twelve pairs of ribs are attached in a hingelike manner posteriorly to the vertebral column. This hingelike attachment allows the chest wall to be mobile during the respiratory cycle. The superior six pairs of ribs are attached anteriorly to the sternum.

The *diaphragm*, the primary muscle of respiration, is composed of two dome-shaped hemidiaphragms that are

Anterior view of thorax

attached to the lower edge of the rib cage. The right hemidiaphragm sits higher than the left. The diaphragm forms the inferior "floor" of the thorax. During inspiration, the diaphragm flattens and descends toward the abdomen. During expiration, it relaxes and ascends to its resting, dome-shaped configuration.

The *external intercostal muscles* are also involved in respiration. These muscles, located between the ribs and innervated by the intercostal nerves, contract during inspiration to stabilize, elevate, and expand the rib cage.

The *accessory muscles of respiration* — the sternocleidomastoid, scalene, trapezius, and rhomboid muscles — are involved in labored or forceful breathing. The sternocleidomastoid muscle elevates the sternum, increasing the anterior-to-posterior chest diameter. The scalene muscles elevate and fix the first two ribs. The trapezius and rhomboid muscles are activated during respiration but probably have no effect on forceful inspiration. The contraction of external intercostal muscles may also be obvious in extremely labored breathing.

Abdominal muscles usually do not participate actively in relaxed breathing but play an important role during forceful expiratory efforts, such as coughing or sneezing. The internal intercostal muscles also contract forcefully during expiration.

Normal breathing

During inspiration, the diaphragm and external intercostal muscles are activated. Diaphragmatic contraction flattens the domed diaphragm and expands the lower rib cage, forcing the abdominal contents downward and out, thus increasing the longitudinal lung size. External intercostal muscle contraction stabilizes the rib cage and moves it outward and upward. The posterior cricoarytenoid muscle contracts to open the glottis. As the thorax expands, intrapleural pressures become subatmospheric, resulting in lung expansion and decreased intrapulmonary pressures. Inspired air flows from higher atmospheric pressure into the airways. At the end of inspiration, diaphragmatic movement declines and the air inflow gradually slows.

During expiration, the thorax and the elastic recoil force of the lungs return to their resting positions, increasing intrapleural pressures. This increased pressure forces air to flow out of the lower and upper airways. At the end of expiration, during quiet breathing, all muscles are relaxed and the diaphragm has returned to its resting position.

Distribution of ventilation and blood flow

During normal breathing in the upright position, air movement (ventilation) is greatest in the lung bases or dependent lung regions. Because of the pull of gravity, the alveoli in the lung bases collapse to a smaller size during expiration than do the alveoli in the lung apices. During inspiration, the alveoli in the lung bases open more easily, causing ventilation in the bases to be greater than in the apices.

Blood perfusion in the lungs is also gravity-dependent; the dependent lung regions receive a larger proportion of the cardiac output than the nondependent regions. When the patient is in the upright position, blood flow patterns in the apices are usually different from those in the bases. In the lung apices, alveolar (atmospheric) pressures exceed capillary hydrostatic pressure, and the capillaries remain partially collapsed during quiet breathing; this results in limited blood flow. In the lung bases, pulmonary arterial and venous hydrostatic pressures exceed atmospheric pressure, and the capillaries remain open throughout quiet breathing; this results in proportionately more blood flow to the lung bases than to the apices.

Diaphragm during inspiration

Diaphragm

Diaphragm during expiration

Diaphragm

Postural changes affect the distribution of ventilation and blood flow throughout the lungs. In the supine position, the apices and bases receive equal amounts of air and blood flow. In the lateral position, dependent lung regions receive more air and blood flow than nondependent regions.

The tracheobronchial tree's dimensions and shape also affect the airflow pattern. During inspiration, air velocity and the airflow rate decrease as the cross-sectional airway area increases. Consequently, the larger airways conduct the same volume of air as do the more numerous smaller airways. This means that inspired air travels 100 times faster in the trachea than it does in the terminal bronchi.

Beyond the terminal bronchi, the forward movement of air is minimal. In the terminal bronchioles, diffusion is the primary method of air movement. The mean airflow velocity during inspiration is approximately 100 m/second in the trachea, but less than 1 cm/second in the terminal bronchioles.

Auscultatory areas

Thoracic structures and landmarks

Accurate interpretation of breath sounds depends on a systematic approach to auscultation; it also requires the ability to describe the location of abnormal findings in relation to bony structures and anatomic landmark lines.

Breath sounds are auscultated over the anterior chest wall surface, the lateral chest wall surfaces, and the posterior chest wall surface.

Anterior chest wall surface

The lung apices extend approximately ¼" to 1½" (2 to 4 cm) above the clavicles. The trachea bifurcates at the level of the sternal angle, the junction between the manubrium and the body of the sternum. The ribs and intercostal spaces provide precise horizontal landmarks to describe the location of breath sounds; the second rib and second intercostal space serve as reference points.

Vertical landmark lines on the anterior chest wall surface include the midclavicular lines and the midsternal line. The right and left midclavicular lines extend downward from the center of each clavicle. The midsternal line bisects the sternum. The right lung base crosses the sixth

Anterior thoracic structures and landmark lines

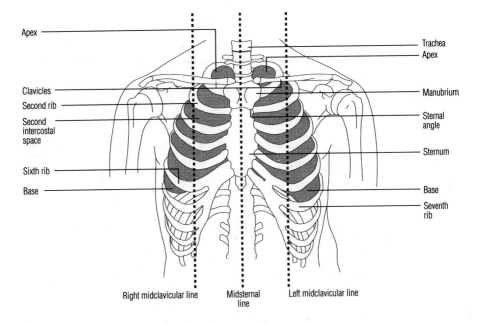

rib at the right midclavicular line, and the left lung base crosses the seventh rib at the left midclavicular line.

Lateral chest wall surfaces

The lateral chest wall surfaces are also divided using landmark lines. The anterior axillary line extends downward from the anterior axillary fold, the midaxillary line extends downward from the apex of the axilla, and the posterior axillary line extends downward from the posterior axillary fold.

Posterior chest wall surface

Bony structures underlying the posterior chest wall surface also provide landmarks to locate breath sounds. The scapulae's inferior borders, located at about the same level as the seventh rib, serve as reference points. The numbered thoracic vertebrae provide horizontal landmarks.

Landmark lines on the posterior chest wall surface provide vertical reference points. The midscapular lines extend downward from the inferior angle of each scapula, and the vertebral line extends downward over the vertebrae.

Right lateral landmark lines

1. Posterior axillary line
2. Midaxillary line
3. Anterior axillary line

Posterior thoracic structures and landmark lines

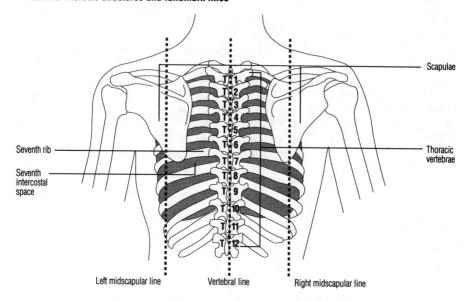

Auscultatory techniques

Using the stethoscope

The stethoscope allows you to hear breath sounds transmitted through the chest wall. Most stethoscopes have a diaphragm and a bell, with one or two tubes leading to the binaural headpiece and earpieces. The diaphragm is used to listen for high-pitched breath sounds; the bell is used to listen for low-pitched breath sounds. Applying the stethoscope firmly to the chest wall amplifies high-frequency sounds. However, if too much pressure is applied when using the bell, the stretched skin functions as a diaphragm and filters out low-pitched sounds.

The stethoscope tubing should be no longer than 10″ to 12″ (25 to 30 cm). It should be tightly attached to the binaural headpiece and the stethoscope body to prevent air leakage, which could result in the loss of sound energy. The earpieces must be securely attached to the binaural headpiece, which removes extraneous noise from the environment, to avoid any sound loss. They should fit tightly and should be placed into the ears in an anterior direction so that they conform to the direction of the ear canals.

Listening to breath sounds

Breath sounds have a wide range of sound frequencies, many near the lower threshold of human hearing. Consequently, the environment for auscultation should be as quiet as possible so that you can hear breath sounds clearly and distinctly. Close the door to the room and eliminate extraneous noises and conversations; turn off televisions and radios. You'll need to develop good concentration skills so that noises from such devices as I.V. pumps, oxygen delivery systems, and ventilators do not interfere with auscultation.

During auscultation, press the diaphragm of the stethoscope firmly against the patient's chest wall over the intercostal spaces. Try not to listen directly over bone. Never listen through clothing, which impedes or alters sound transmission. Avoid other extraneous sounds such as those caused by the stethoscope rubbing against bed rails or other objects.

AUSCULTATION TIP If the patient has a very hairy chest, lightly dampen the chest and hold the stethoscope firmly against the skin to minimize the crackling noises produced by the hair.

Auscultatory sequence

The auscultatory sequence for the posterior chest wall surface includes 10 different sites. (See *Posterior auscultatory sequence*.) The first site is above the left scapula over the lung apex. From there, the auscultatory sequence follows a pattern that progresses downward from the lung

Posterior auscultatory sequence

Anterior auscultatory sequence

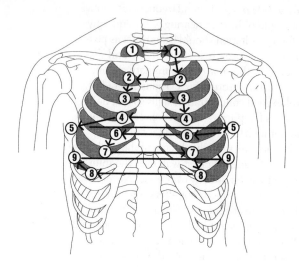

apices to the bases. This pattern covers the entire posterior chest wall surface and includes a comparison of sounds heard over the same auscultatory site over both the right and left lungs. Sites 5, 7, and 10 are located over the lateral chest wall surfaces.

The anterior chest wall auscultatory sequence includes nine sites and follows the same pattern as the posterior chest wall sequence. The pattern also includes sites over the lateral chest wall surfaces.

Comparing breath sounds

If the patient is alert and healthy, begin auscultation with the patient sitting upright and leaning slightly forward. Position yourself behind the patient. Ask the patient to breathe through an open mouth, slightly deeper than usual, through several respiratory cycles. (*Note:* If the patient is extremely dyspneic, don't ask him to take deeper breaths. In this case, begin auscultating for breath sounds at the bilateral lung bases.) Place the diaphragm of the stethoscope over the left lung apex, and listen for at least one complete respiratory cycle. Then move the diaphragm to the same site over the right lung. Compare the breath sounds heard over these same locations. Continue in this manner, making contralateral comparisons at each auscultatory site.

After you have auscultated the entire posterior chest wall and parts of the lateral chest walls, move to the front of the patient. Have the patient place his arms at his sides and breathe through an open mouth, slightly deeper than usual, as you listen to breath sounds over the anterior chest wall. You can obtain additional information about tracheal sounds by auscultating over the sternum, larynx, and mouth.

◎ **AUSCULTATION TIP** You may roll comatose, critically ill, or bedridden patients from one side to another to auscultate dependent lung regions. Listen initially over dependent lung regions because gravity-dependent secretions or fluids may produce abnormal sounds that sometimes disappear when the patient is turned, breathes deeply, or coughs.

◤ *POSTTEST*

1. What is the primary function of the respiratory system?
2. Name the anatomic structures of the upper airway.
3. Name the three sections of the pharynx.
4. Name the anatomic structures of the lower airway.
5. Where is the trachea located?
6. Describe the anatomy of the lower airway from the mainstem bronchi to the alveoli.
7. What is anatomic dead space?
8. What are the functions of the airways' mucus layer and cilia?
9. How are the lungs separated into lobes?
10. Where are the lung's apex and base located?
11. What are the three types of cells found in the alveoli?
12. What is surfactant and where is it found?
13. What roles do the parasympathetic and sympathetic nervous systems have in the lower airways?
14. Describe the pulmonary circulation in the lungs.
15. Describe the bronchial circulation in the lungs.
16. What are the pleurae?
17. What is the thorax's function during breathing?
18. What is the primary muscle of respiration and how does it contribute to breathing?
19. How do the external intercostal muscles contribute to breathing?
20. Name the accessory muscles of respiration, and describe their role in breathing.
21. Describe normal breathing.
22. How are ventilation and blood flow distributed in the lungs?

23. Describe how postural changes affect ventilation and blood flow distribution.
24. How do the tracheobronchial tree's dimensions and shape influence airflow patterns?
25. Name the anatomic structures and landmark lines on the anterior chest wall surface.
26. Name the anatomic structures and landmark lines on the lateral chest wall surfaces.
27. Name the anatomic structures and landmark lines on the posterior chest wall surface.
28. What are the functions of the diaphragm and bell of the stethoscope?
29. How is the stethoscope used to auscultate for breath sounds?
30. Describe the sequence used during auscultation to compare breath sounds.

2

Introduction to breath sounds

▶ *PRETEST*
1. How are breath sounds produced?
2. What is airway dynamics?
3. Name three different airflow patterns.
4. How is the frequency of vibrations measured?
5. Explain the concept of sound damping.
6. Explain the concept of impedance matching.
7. What are egophony, bronchophony, and whispered pectoriloquy?
8. What are adventitious sounds?
9. Name the four characteristics of breath sounds that should be documented in a patient's record.

Breath sound production

Three types of sounds are heard during auscultation — normal breath sounds, abnormal breath sounds (including voice sounds), and adventitious sounds. Breath sounds are produced by airflow patterns, by associated pressure changes within the airways, and by solid tissue vibrations. Both normal and abnormal breath sounds have certain recognizable characteristics. Their amplitude and intensity are believed to be affected by airflow patterns, regional lung volume or distribution of ventilation, body position, and the sound production site.

The sounds are normally diminished and filtered when they are transmitted through air-filled alveoli, fluid accumulations in the pleura, and solid structures such as bone.

The sites where normal breath sounds originate are not clearly defined. For example, sounds heard over the

19

trachea and large airways are characterized as loud and tubular (hollow) with a long expiratory phase. These sounds are thought to reflect the turbulent airflow patterns in the first divisions of the large airways.

Sounds heard over other chest wall areas are softer and have a shorter expiratory phase. These sounds may also be produced by turbulent airflow in the first few divisions of the large airways; however, the fact that these sounds vary with changing airflow rates and distribution of ventilation in the lungs suggests that they are produced in the peripheral airways. Also, inspiratory sounds may be produced in the peripheral airways, and expiratory sounds may be produced in the larger airways. Breath sounds are not produced in the terminal bronchioles because of minimal airflow rates.

Disease processes that alter the airway or airflow dynamics produce abnormal breath sounds or adventitious sounds. These sounds are generated by the vibration of solid structures, by airflow through narrowed airways, or by abrupt changes in airway pressures.

Airway dynamics

An airway's stability depends on the interaction among the elastic properties of the lung tissue, the intrapulmonary airways, and the pressures — both internal and external — exerted on the airways. During the respiratory cycle, a pressure gradient exists across the airway wall and between the trachea and alveoli. As the chest expands during inspiration, intrapleural pressure falls. At the same time, the lung's elastic recoil increases, exerting traction on airway walls. This traction increases the airways' diameter and decreases the resistance to airflow. The pressure gradient between the alveolar and atmospheric pressures increases, driving air through the airways toward the alveoli.

Intrapleural pressure and alveolar elastic recoil pressures drive expiratory airflow. At the beginning of expiration, intrapleural pressure and the alveolar recoil force cause the alveolar pressures to rise and push the air through the airways and out through the mouth. Air pressures fall as the air flows through the airways from the alveoli to the mouth. A point is reached, particularly during forceful expiration, when intrapleural and intrapulmonary pressures are equal; this normally occurs in the segmental bronchi and is called the *equal pressure point*. Downstream from this point, pressures outside of the airways can compress and further narrow the airways, causing increased resistance to airflow.

Airflow patterns
Variations in airflow patterns are affected by the intricate network of branching airways, the various airway diameters, and the potential for irregular airway wall surfaces within the tracheobronchial tree.

Turbulent airflow
During rapid, or turbulent, airflow, air molecules move randomly, colliding against airway walls and each other.

They may move across or against the general direction of airflow. The colliding air molecules produce rapid pressure changes within the airway, and these rapid pressure changes produce sounds. Turbulent airflow occurs in the trachea, mainstem bronchi, and other larger airways.

Vortices
As airflow is forced to change directions abruptly in the branching airways, the airstream separates into layers and moves at different velocities. The shearing force of high velocity airstreams, along with slower airstreams, precipitates opposing circular airflows, or vortices. This airflow pattern generates sounds as the flow of air carries the vortices downstream.

Laminar airflow
In the terminal or small airways and respiratory bronchioles, airflow is slow and laminar. No abrupt changes in pressure or airway wall movements occur to generate sound. Consequently, air movement in these areas produces no sound.

Mechanical vibrations
Breath sounds are also produced by mechanical vibrations of solid tissue. These vibrations travel through the different media of air, fluid, or tissue at varying speeds. Their frequency, intensity, and duration can be measured.

Frequency, measured in hertz (Hz), refers to the number of vibrations occurring per unit of time. Different

Turbulent airflow

Airway walls

Vortices

Airway walls

Laminar airflow

Airway walls

frequencies produce the different sounds heard during auscultation. In the clinical setting, the term pitch is used to describe sound frequency. High-pitched sounds have higher frequencies; low-pitched sounds have lower frequencies.

Intensity, the loudness or softness of the vibrations producing breath sounds, can be measured electronically by recording amplitude. Intensity is affected by the type of vibrating structure producing the sound, the distance the sound travels, and the transmission pathway.

The *duration* of the vibrations that produce breath sounds can be measured in milliseconds (msec). However, the human ear perceives sounds during auscultation as long or short and as continuous or discontinuous.

Sound damping

Body structures or cavities that produce resonance will selectively transmit or amplify breath sounds that are similar in frequency and will absorb, or damp, those with other frequencies. Breath sounds arising from the same location in the lung have a higher pitch when heard at the mouth or over the trachea than when heard over the chest wall. This change in pitch occurs because high-pitched breath sounds are absorbed as they are transmitted through the lungs and thorax.

Voice sounds are also affected by damping. The resonant qualities of the mouth, nasopharynx, paranasal sinuses, and chest cavity contribute to the pitch and intensity of voice sounds.

Impedance matching

Breath and voice sounds are normally damped when they're transmitted through air, fluid, and tissue. But when these sounds are transmitted sequentially through media with different acoustical properties, the sounds' vibrations are filtered and reflected at the interface of the different media. The amount of filtering that takes place depends on the media's impedance (resistance to sound transmission).

When two media are matched according to acoustical properties, sound is transmitted effectively. For example, consolidated areas enhance the transmission of breath sounds to the chest wall. This happens because the consolidating substance, an inflammatory exudate, collects in alveoli, replacing air with dense lung tissue. Consequently, the fluid-filled, airless lung tissue and the chest wall are acoustically well matched, and breath sounds are transmitted more easily.

On the other hand, the transmission of breath and voice sounds through either tissue or fluid between inflated lung segments and the chest wall results in an impedance mismatch. The vibrations of the sounds are significantly filtered and reflected back to their source by the pleurae. Diseases that increase the impedance mismatch, such as a large pleural effusion or empyema, diminish breath sound intensity. Obesity is also associated with diminished breath sounds because of the increased distance between the stethoscope and the lungs.

◉ **AUSCULTATION TIP** For better results when auscultating an obese patient's lungs, ask him to take deep breaths while sitting upright or standing.

Terminology

Classifying breath sounds

Normal breath sounds are classified as tracheal and mainstem bronchi sounds and normal breath sounds heard over other chest wall areas. The tracheal and mainstem bronchi sounds, produced by turbulent airflow, are loud and can be heard throughout inspiration and expiration over the trachea and mainstem bronchi. (♦1____) Normal breath sounds heard over other chest wall areas are faint and can be heard throughout inspiration and at the beginning of expiration. (♦2____) (See Chapter 3 for a further discussion of normal breath sound terminology.)

Many clinicians think bronchovesicular breath sounds represent a third classification of normal sounds. These sounds are heard over areas between the mainstem bronchi and the smaller airways; their pitch and duration are midway between those of tracheal and mainstem bronchi breath sounds and normal breath sounds heard over other chest wall areas. (♦3____) Bronchovesicular sounds are heard during inspiration and expiration for equal amounts of time.

Classifying voice sounds

Voice sounds are vibrations produced by speech that are transmitted to the chest wall through the tracheobronchial tree. Voice sounds are classified as bronchophony, egophony, and whispered pectoriloquy.

Voice sounds auscultated over the chest wall are called *bronchophony.* In a healthy individual, bronchophony is similar to voice sounds heard through the neck. (♦4_____) Voice sounds transmitted through the chest wall that have selectively amplified higher frequencies are called *egophony.* (♦5_____) High-pitched whispered sounds transmitted through airless, consolidated lung tissue are called *whispered pectoriloquy.* (♦6_____)

Classifying adventitious sounds

Adventitious sounds are added sounds that are heard with normal and abnormal breath sounds. They are divided into two classifications — crackles and wheezes — that are further classified by duration and pitch. (See Chapter 7 for a further discussion of adventitious breath sound terminology.)

Documenting auscultation findings

Careful documentation of auscultation findings is necessary to determine if sounds heard have changed over time. This requires the same systematic approach used during auscultation. First, determine the location, intensity, duration, and pitch of each sound during auscultation, and then document these characteristics in the patient's record.

Document sound *location* by describing anatomic thoracic landmarks and indicating the anterior, posterior, or lateral chest wall surface where the sound is heard.

You can also document location by using the lung bases or apices as reference points. Also document whether the sounds are heard bilaterally (over both lungs) or unilaterally (over one lung).

Sound *intensity* is described subjectively, using such terms as loud, soft, absent, diminished, or distant.

Sound *duration* refers to the sound's timing within the respiratory cycle — that is, whether it is heard during inspiration, expiration, or both. Timing can be described as early, late, or throughout.

Sound *pitch* is usually described as high or low. Documenting pitch is more important when wheezes or crackles have been noted during auscultation because pitch helps differentiate the underlying disease process.

A typical documentation example might read: "Late inspiratory fine crackles were heard over the right base posteriorly along the midscapular line, and coarse crackles were heard throughout inspiration and expiration over the left apex anteriorly near the midclavicular line." Such a description provides the reader with valuable information about any adventitious sounds heard during auscultation.

◤ POSTTEST

1. How are breath sounds produced?
2. Briefly describe the differences between breath sounds heard over the trachea and mainstem bronchi and those heard over other chest wall areas.
3. What role do pressure gradients have in breathing?
4. Describe how intrapleural pressure and alveolar elastic recoil pressures serve as the driving pressure for expiratory flow.
5. What influences airflow patterns?
6. Describe turbulent airflow.
7. Describe vortices.
8. Describe laminar airflow.
9. What is meant by frequency, intensity, and duration of breath sounds?
10. Explain the concept of sound damping.
11. Explain the concept of impedance matching.
12. What happens to impedance matching when the lungs become air- or fluid-filled?
13. Compare and contrast tracheal and mainstem bronchi breath sounds with normal breath sounds heard over other chest wall areas.
14. What are bronchovesicular breath sounds?
15. Define the terms bronchophony, egophony, and whispered pectoriloquy.

16. What are adventitious sounds?
17. Name the four characteristics used to describe breath sounds.
18. What terms are used to describe sound intensity?
19. What terms are used to describe sound duration?
20. What terms are used to describe sound pitch?

Normal Breath Sounds

3

Breath sounds heard in healthy individuals

▶️ *PRETEST*
1. What are normal breath sounds?
2. How do normal breath sounds originate?
3. What affects normal breath sound characteristics?
4. What is the significance of breath sounds heard at the mouth?

Anatomy and physiology

In 1816, René Laënnec classified normal breath sounds as either pulmonary or bronchial. He later substituted the term *vesicular* for *pulmonary* because he believed the sounds were produced in the terminal airways and alveoli. In 1978, P. Forgacs proposed that normal breath sounds be classified as tracheal and mainstem bronchi sounds and normal breath sounds heard over other chest wall areas.

Normal breath sounds are broadly defined as breathing heard through the chest wall of a healthy person. They are classified as bronchial, vesicular, and bronchovesicular. Three variables affect the normal sounds heard during auscultation: the distance between the source of the sound and the chest wall, the path of sound transmission, and the sound's location. Normal breath sounds are produced by airflow patterns, by associated pressure changes within the airways, and by solid tissue vibrations.

Normal breath sounds heard over large airways are produced by turbulent airflow in those airways. They're loudest when auscultated over the trachea on the anterior chest wall surface next to the sternum. As air travels through the airways beyond the segmental bronchi, these normally high-pitched sounds become diminished because they are filtered by the chest wall, pleurae, and air-

Auscultatory sites for tracheal and mainstem bronchi breath sounds

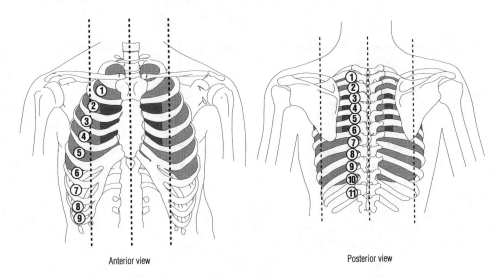

Anterior view   Posterior view

filled lung tissue. The normal breath sounds heard over most of the chest wall surface are soft and low-pitched; they are softer and shorter during expiration than during inspiration.

Tracheal and mainstem bronchi breath sounds

Normal breath sounds heard over the trachea and mainstem bronchi (bronchial breath sounds) are produced by turbulent airflow patterns and are described as tubular (hollow) and harsh. Inspired and expired air travels easily through these large airways.

A brief pause may be heard at the end of inspiration, and expiration is longer than inspiration. The inspiratory-expiratory (I:E) ratio is 1:2 to 1:3. The sound frequency distribution of these breath sounds is 200 to 2,000 Hz. (♦7____)

Tracheal and mainstem bronchi (bronchial) breath sounds are heard over the chest wall on either side of the sternum from the second intercostal space to the fourth intercostal space anteriorly and along the vertebral column from the third intercostal space to the sixth intercostal space posteriorly. These sounds have a variable pitch and a loud intensity heard best with the diaphragm of the

Airway area producing tracheal and mainstem bronchi breath sounds

1. Trachea
2. Right mainstem bronchus
3. Left mainstem bronchus

Auscultatory sites for normal breath sounds heard over other chest wall areas

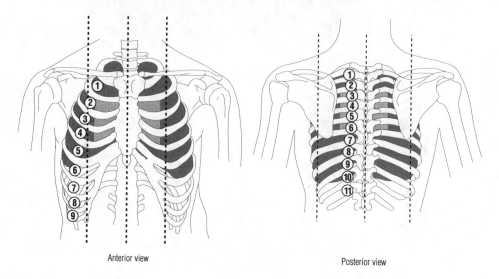

Anterior view

Posterior view

stethoscope; they're heard throughout inspiration and expiration. (♦8____)

Normal breath sounds heard over other chest wall areas

Normal breath sounds (also known as vesicular breath sounds) transmitted through lung tissue and the chest wall are produced by changes in airflow patterns. These normal sounds are quieter than tracheal and mainstem bronchi sounds. Inspiration is heard clearly, and expiration immediately follows inspiration but quickly fades as airflow rates rapidly decline and turbulent airflow is directed toward the central airways. The I:E ratio is 3:1 to 4:1. The sound frequency distribution of these normal breath sounds is 200 to 600 Hz. (♦9____)

Airway areas producing normal breath sounds heard over other chest wall areas

Variations in breath sound intensity

Bronchovesicular breath sounds are the third category of breath sounds. They are heard anteriorly and posteriorly over the central large airways. Their pitch and duration are midway between those of the vesicular breath sounds and the bronchial sounds; inspiratory and expiratory phases are equal, with an I:E ratio of 1:1.

The intensity of these normal breath sounds changes during deep inspiration and after maximal expiration. Intensity may also change depending on the lung area being auscultated. For example, if the patient is sitting up during auscultation of the anterior chest wall surface, breath sounds are louder over the apices during early inspiration and become progressively softer as inspiration continues. (♦10____) During auscultation of the posterior lung bases, breath sounds are initially softer and become progressively louder during maximal inspiration.

Variations in intensity are most often related to airflow patterns and to the distribution of ventilation throughout the lungs. During inspiration with the patient in the upright position, air flows initially into the lung apices, then into the lung bases (the dependent areas) after the small airways reopen; therefore, intensity will probably be greater in the apices than in the bases. During normal breathing, this change in intensity may not always be audible.

Variations in intensity that are unrelated to airflow rates or regional ventilation may be heard when comparing symmetrical sites on the chest wall. For example, breath sounds heard over the left lower lobe may vary in intensity with the cardiac cycle. Intensity may increase during systole because ventricular contraction allows the surrounding lung tissue to expand more fully, increasing turbulent airflow to that region and intensifying the inspiratory sounds. Conversely, intensity may decrease during diastole because ventricular expansion of the heart compresses adjacent lung tissue, reducing airflow to that region.

These normal breath sounds are heard throughout the chest anteriorly, posteriorly, and laterally. Their duration varies, depending on their location, but inspiration is usually followed immediately by a shorter expiration. These sounds have a low pitch that can be heard with either the diaphragm or bell of the stethoscope. (♦11____)

Normal breath sounds heard at the mouth

Normal breath sounds can also be heard at the mouth. They are thought to be produced by turbulent airflow occurring below the glottis and before the terminal airways. In healthy individuals, breath sounds at the mouth provide baseline data that can be useful later when evaluating noisy or paradoxically quiet breath sounds.

Airway area producing normal breath sounds heard at mouth

Normal breath sounds heard at the mouth are heard at the lips. Their intensity is as loud and harsh as that of tracheal and mainstem bronchi breath sounds, and their duration is continuous (throughout the respiratory cycle). They have a moderately high pitch.

◀️ POSTTEST

1. Define normal breath sounds.
2. What variables affect normal breath sounds heard during auscultation?
3. How are normal breath sounds produced?
4. Describe tracheal and mainstem bronchi breath sounds.
5. Describe breath sounds heard over other chest wall areas.
6. How do ventilation and airflow rate changes affect breath sound intensity?
7. How do cardiac systole and diastole affect normal breath sound intensity?
8. How are breath sounds heard at the mouth produced?

Abnormal Breath Sounds

4

Bronchial breath sounds

▶❙ *PRETEST*

1. What happens to normal breath sounds when lung density increases?
2. What are bronchial breath sounds?
3. How does consolidation affect breath sounds?
4. How does atelectasis affect breath sounds?
5. How does fibrosis affect breath sounds?

Sound production

When lung tissue between the central airways and the chest wall becomes airless because of conditions that increase lung density, transmission of breath sounds from large airways is enhanced. This happens because very little high-frequency sound is lost through attenuation or filtration. As the lung tissue density increases the impedance between the fluid-filled lung tissue and the pleurae and chest wall, these three media become well matched, which decreases the normal filtering of high-frequency sounds. Consequently, breath sounds are transmitted more readily to the chest wall surface and are louder and more tubular than normal breath sounds heard over the same chest wall area. Expiration is significantly louder and longer than normal. The inspiratory-expiratory (I:E) ratio changes from the normal 3:1 or 4:1 to 1:1 or 1:2. These sounds, called *bronchial breath sounds,* are considered abnormal when found anywhere except anteriorly over the large airways.

Related conditions

Conditions associated with bronchial breath sounds include consolidation, atelectasis, and fibrosis, all of which increase lung tissue density because of fluid accumulation, lung collapse, or fibrotic scarring. Bronchial breath sounds are heard over the affected lung area.

Consolidation

The most common cause of lung tissue consolidation (solidification) is pneumonia, a lung inflammation that can be caused by bacteria, viruses, or chemical insults (such as with aspiration). In this condition, fluid, leukocytes, and erythrocytes accumulate in spaces that are normally air-filled, producing a consolidated area. Clinical findings will vary, depending on the location of the consolidated area and the causative agent. When classic consolidation is present, decreased chest wall movement and a dull percussion note will be apparent over the affected area. Bronchial breath sounds will be heard over a dense, airless *upper* lobe even without a patent bronchus (♦ 12____), because the upper lobe surfaces are in direct contact with the trachea and loud tracheal breath sounds are transmitted directly to the dense, airless upper lobe tissues. In contrast, bronchial breath sounds will be heard over a dense, airless *lower* lobe only when the bronchi are patent, because sound is not transmitted directly to the airless lower lobe tissues.

SOUND CHARACTERISTICS

In a patient with lobar pneumonia with right posterior mid-lung consolidation, bronchial breath sounds are heard over the right posterior midlung field, located over the seventh and eighth intercostal spaces along the vertebral column. (See *Bronchial breath sounds heard over consolidated right posterior midlung,* page 36.) These sounds are high-pitched and have the typical hollow, or tubular, quality of normal central airway breath sounds. They remain audible during both expiration and inspiration, but the expiratory sounds are longer and louder when the patient is sitting up; the I:E ratio is 1:2. These sounds may be auscultated with either the bell or diaphragm of the stethoscope. (♦ 13____)

Atelectasis

Atelectasis, incomplete expansion of a lung area, is typically diagnosed in postoperative or immobile patients and in some patients with bronchiectasis or pneumonia. It is thought to result from prolonged shallow breathing (hypoventilation) or uncleared secretions that become thick, occluding the airway. Because no air enters the distal airways, the segmental or lobar bronchi collapse. If a large airway is occluded, clinical findings will include decreased

Bronchial breath sounds heard over consolidated right posterior midlung

Affected lung area

Posterior auscultatory sites

chest wall movement, a dull percussion note, regional changes in lung volume, and bronchial breath sounds over a dense, airless upper airway. (♦14____) However, decreased chest wall movement and lung volume changes may be very difficult to detect on clinical examination.

ALERT If you hear bronchial breath sounds in upper lobes and absent breath sounds in lower lobes, assume there's a large airway occlusion and provide measures to maintain oxygenation.

SOUND CHARACTERISTICS

Bronchial breath sounds are heard over an atelectatic area when the bronchus is patent. They won't be heard over an atelectatic lower lobe if the bronchus is obstructed.

In an unresponsive patient with a head injury, bronchial breath sounds are heard over the right anterior midlung field, located between the third and fifth intercostal spaces from the midsternal line to just right of the midclavicular line. These sounds are high-pitched and have the typical hollow, or tubular, quality of normal central airway breath sounds. They are audible throughout inspiration and expiration. When the patient is in the supine position, the inspiratory and expiratory sounds are equal in duration and intensity; the I:E ratio is 1:1. These sounds can be heard equally well with either the bell or diaphragm of the stethoscope. (♦15____)

Bronchial breath sounds heard over atelectatic right midlung

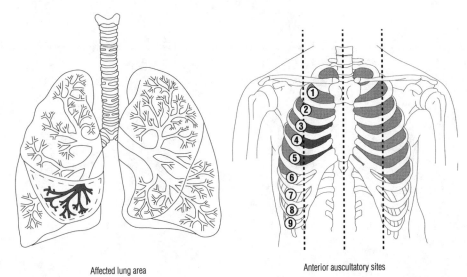

Affected lung area

Anterior auscultatory sites

Fibrosis

Severe fibrosis (abnormal formation of fibrous connective tissue) may produce bronchial breath sounds that are usually heard over the lower lung regions. Interstitial pulmonary fibrosis is a pathologic change caused by many chronic inflammatory diseases that produce diffuse lung injury. Some common causes of pulmonary fibrosis are chronic smoke inhalation and chronic exposure to asbestos or silica. The breath sounds heard over fibrotic areas are similar to those heard over atelectatic areas. (♦16____)

Lung area affected by asbestosis

SOUND CHARACTERISTICS

In a patient with asbestosis, bronchial breath sounds are heard anteriorly and posteriorly over both lung bases.

Anteriorly, this area extends from the midsternal line to the right and left of the anterior axillary lines over the fifth and sixth intercostal spaces; posteriorly, it extends from the vertebral line to the right and left of the posterior axillary lines over the seventh, eighth, ninth, and tenth intercostal spaces. (See *Auscultatory sites for asbestosis in lung bases,* page 38.)

Because the bronchi are patent, bronchial breath sounds heard over fibrotic areas have the typical hollow, or tubular, quality of normal central airway breath sounds. They are audible throughout inspiration and expiration. When the patient is in the upright position, the breath

Auscultatory sites for asbestosis in lung bases

Anterior view

Posterior view

sounds become progressively louder during inspiration and become both louder and longer during expiration; the I:E ratio is 1:1 to 1:2. These bronchial breath sounds are high-pitched and are heard equally well with either the diaphragm or bell of the stethoscope. (♦17____)

◀ *POSTTEST*

1. What happens when lung tissue becomes airless because of conditions that increase lung density?
2. Why are breath sounds enhanced over an area of increased lung density?
3. Name three conditions associated with bronchial breath sounds.
4. What clinical findings are typically associated with consolidation?
5. What role does a patent bronchus have in the transmission of breath sounds to the apex and base of the lung?
6. Describe the characteristics of bronchial breath sounds heard over a consolidated area.
7. What causes atelectasis?
8. Describe the characteristics of bronchial breath sounds heard over an atelectatic area.
9. Describe the characteristics of bronchial breath sounds heard over a fibrotic area.

5

Abnormal voice sounds

▶❙ *PRETEST*
1. How are normal voice sounds produced?
2. Name three voice sounds.
3. How do voice sounds change over areas of dense, airless lung tissue?
4. What specific words or letters is the patient asked to repeat to detect changes in bronchophony, whispered pectoriloquy, and egophony?
5. What auscultatory findings are associated with consolidation?

Sound production

Voice sounds are produced by vibrations of the vocal cords as air from the lungs passes over them. The resonance of the mouth, nasopharynx, and paranasal sinuses helps to amplify these sounds. When voice sounds pass through normally inflated, air-filled lungs, vowel tones, which contain many high-frequency sounds, are diminished and filtered. Like other high-frequency sounds, voice sounds are also selectively reflected back toward the lung tissue at the pleurae. Consequently, transmitted voice sounds are normally heard as a low-pitched, unintelligible mumble over healthy lung and pleural surfaces because most of the vowels are filtered out; conversely, they are heard distinctly over consolidated or atelectatic lung tissue areas because less filtering takes place, enhancing transmission.

Three types
The three types of voice sounds are bronchophony, whispered pectoriloquy, and egophony.

Auscultatory sites for bronchophony heard over consolidated left upper lobe

Anterior view

Posterior view

Consolidated lung area producing bronchophony in left upper lobe

Bronchophony

Bronchophony is the clear, distinct, intelligible voice sound heard over dense, airless lung tissue. (♦18____) Dense, airless lung tissue transmits high-frequency vowel sounds more easily because of impedance matching. Also, consolidation increases vocal resonance, which allows the clear transmission of voice sounds to the chest wall. Bronchophony is heard over dense, airless *upper* lobes because the upper lobe surfaces are in direct contact with the trachea, leading to direct transmission of tracheal breath sounds. In contrast, bronchophony is heard over dense, airless *lower* lobes only when the bronchi are patent because a direct path of sound transmission to the lower lobes does not exist.

SOUND CHARACTERISTICS

Bronchophony can be heard anywhere over the anterior, lateral, and posterior chest wall surfaces. It is commonly heard over dense, airless lung tissue in the upper lobes, such as a consolidated area. In a patient with left upper lobe pneumonia, intelligible voice sounds are heard over both the anterior and posterior chest wall surfaces. The anterior area is located between the space above the clavicle and the second intercostal space from the midsternal line to the left of the midclavicular line. The posterior area is located between the first and third intercostal

Auscultatory sites for whispered pectoriloquy heard over atelectatic left lower lobe

Anterior view

Posterior view

spaces from the vertebral line toward the left midscapular line.

The patient is asked to repeat the words "ninety-nine" several times. Over healthy lung tissue, the words are unintelligible (♦19____); over a consolidated area, however, the high-frequency sounds are easily understood as words. (♦20____)

Whispered pectoriloquy

Whispered pectoriloquy is the clear, distinct, intelligible whispered voice sound heard over airless, consolidated, or atelectatic lung tissue. In a healthy person, normal lung tissue filters the high frequencies of whispered vowel sounds, making them unintelligible during auscultation. In a patient with consolidation or atelectasis, these same whispered vowel sounds are transmitted to the chest wall surface without much filtering of high frequencies and can be heard clearly with the stethoscope. (♦21____)

SOUND CHARACTERISTICS

Whispered pectoriloquy can be heard anywhere over the anterior or posterior chest wall surfaces over dense, airless lung tissue, typically over an area of consolidation or atelectasis. In a postoperative patient with left lower lobe atelectasis and a patent bronchus, intelligible voice sounds are heard over the anterior and posterior chest wall sur-

Atelectatic lung area producing whispered pectoriloquy in left lower lobe

Consolidated lung area producing egophony in right lower lobe

Auscultatory sites for egophony heard over consolidated right lower lobe

Right lateral view

faces. The anterior area is located over the fifth and sixth intercostal spaces from the midsternal line to the midaxillary line. The posterior area is located over the eighth, ninth, and tenth intercostal spaces from the vertebral line to the midaxillary line.

The patient is asked to whisper the words "one-two-three" several times. Over healthy lung tissue, the words are unintelligible (♦22____); over the atelectatic area, the high-frequency vowel sounds are easily understood as words. (♦23____)

Egophony

Egophony, a voice sound that has a nasal or bleating quality when heard over the chest wall (♦24____), is produced over consolidated and atelectatic areas because impedance matching enhances breath sound transmission in such areas. It is also detectable over the upper border of large pleural effusions.

SOUND CHARACTERISTICS

Egophony can be heard anywhere over the anterior, posterior, or lateral chest wall surfaces over a consolidated or atelectatic area. In a patient with right lower lobe pneumonia, egophony is heard over the lateral chest wall surface. This area is located over the fifth and sixth intercostal spaces between the anterior axillary line and the midaxillary line.

The patient is asked to repeat the letter "E" several times. Over healthy lung tissue, the letter sounds as it normally does (♦25____); over the consolidated area, it sounds like "A-aay" and has a high-pitched, nasal quality. (♦26____)

Constellation of findings

A constellation of auscultatory findings — bronchial breath sounds, bronchophony, whispered pectoriloquy, and egophony — is typical in patients with consolidation. Bronchophony may be easier to hear when bronchial breath sounds are pronounced and consolidation is present in only one lobe or lung. Whispered pectoriloquy is often discernible over atelectatic lung segments or areas of patchy consolidation where bronchial sounds or bronchophony is not completely audible.

▌◀ *POSTTEST*

1. How are voice sounds produced?
2. Describe voice sounds heard over normal lung and pleural surfaces.
3. What happens to voice sounds heard over a consolidated area or an atelectatic area?
4. How does bronchophony change over dense, airless lung tissue?
5. What role does a patent bronchus have in transmitting bronchophony to the lung's apex and base?
6. Describe bronchophony's characteristics.
7. What words is the patient asked to repeat to detect changes in bronchophony?
8. How does whispered pectoriloquy change over dense, airless lung tissue?
9. Describe whispered pectoriloquy's characteristics.
10. What words is the patient asked to repeat to detect changes in whispered pectoriloquy?
11. How is egophony produced over dense, airless lung tissue?
12. Describe egophony's characteristics.
13. What letter is the patient asked to repeat to detect changes in egophony?
14. What constellation of auscultatory findings is typical in patients with consolidation?

6

Absent and diminished breath sounds

▶️ *PRETEST*

1. What conditions are associated with diminished or absent breath sounds?
2. How does each of these conditions cause diminished or absent breath sounds?
3. Explain the concepts of impedance mismatch and filtering.
4. Does lung hyperinflation cause diminished or absent breath sounds?
5. How does positive end-expiratory pressure change normal breath sound characteristics?
6. Does obesity change normal breath sound characteristics?

Sound production

Breath sounds are diminished or eliminated by conditions that limit airflow into lung segments. Slow inspiratory airflow rates decrease breath sound amplitude because less air movement occurs, resulting in less turbulent airflow.

Diminished or absent breath sounds can also occur when breath sounds are reflected at the visceral and parietal pleurae because of an impedance mismatch. A mismatch occurs when sounds are transmitted through two types of media with significantly different acoustical properties. For example, when breath sounds, which are normally transmitted through aerated lung tissue, are transmitted through a collection of fluid or air in the pleural space, sound transmission is halted or filtered. The same acoustical mismatch also occurs in patients with increased chest wall thickness. For example, in obese patients, breath sounds are diminished as they're transmitted through a layer of fat.

Lobar bronchus obstruction

Obstruction

Absent breath sounds

Related conditions

Conditions associated with absent or diminished breath sounds include shallow breathing, diaphragmatic paralysis, severe airway obstruction, pneumothorax, pleural effusion, hyperinflated lungs, and obesity. The use of positive end-expiratory pressure (PEEP) during assisted ventilation also is associated with diminished breath sounds.

Shallow breathing

During normal breathing in the upright position, a certain amount of air flows through the airways during inspiration and expiration; the distribution of ventilation is greater in dependent lung regions because more respiratory movement occurs. During shallow breathing, less respiratory movement occurs; consequently, less air flows through the airways during inspiration and expiration. Because of this reduced airflow, turbulence is decreased and breath sounds are diminished. (♦27____) These softer sounds may be heard over the anterior, posterior, and lateral chest wall surfaces. Shallow breathing occurs when pain limits depth of respiration, as in patients with rib fractures, postoperative patients, and patients whose level of consciousness is depressed from central nervous system injuries or drug overdoses.

Decreased turbulent airflow in shallow breathing

Airway walls

Diaphragmatic paralysis

During inspiration in a healthy person, contraction of the dome-shaped diaphragm expands the lower rib cage, forcing the abdominal contents downward and out and increasing

Mainstem bronchus obstruction

Obstruction

Absent breath sounds

longitudinal lung size. Thoracic expansion lowers intrapulmonary pressure, which allows air to flow into the airways.

When the diaphragm becomes paralyzed, as might happen with injury to the phrenic nerves, it no longer participates in normal breathing. The internal and external intercostal muscles, which also have a role in normal breathing, must take over the work of breathing. With only the chest wall muscles initiating the respiratory cycle, ventilation of the lung bases may be limited, resulting in diminished breath sounds. These diminished sounds may be heard over the anterior, posterior, and lateral chest wall surfaces. (♦28____)

ALERT In the patient with diaphragmatic paralysis, who has greatly diminished breath sounds, assess for respiratory distress and prepare for intubation and mechanical ventilation.

Airway obstruction
Airways must be patent for air to flow through them during inspiration and expiration. If a lobar or segmental bronchus becomes obstructed, as in a patient who has aspirated a foreign object or one with a large mucus plug, airflow ceases distal to the obstruction; therefore, breath sounds will be absent over the area distal to the obstruction. If a mainstem bronchus is obstructed, breath sounds will be absent throughout the entire affected lung. (See *Mainstem bronchus obstruction.*)

Pneumothorax affecting left lateral lung field

Affected lung area

Left lateral auscultatory sites

ALERT When a patient has aspirated a foreign object and continues to cough, don't intervene — allow the patient to cough up the object if possible.

Pneumothorax

A pneumothorax is the accumulation of air in the normally airless pleural space because of a tear in either the visceral or parietal pleura. Breath sounds heard over a pneumothorax are significantly diminished or absent because of acoustical mismatching of the air-filled lung and the collection of air in the pleural space. (♦29____)

The degree of change in breath sounds depends on the size of the pneumothorax. A small pneumothorax may not alter the breath sound intensity enough to be heard during auscultation; it may, however, be apparent on a chest X-ray. A large pneumothorax significantly diminishes breath sounds or permits no sound transmission, causing absent breath sounds. Typical pneumothorax characteristics include sharp, stabbing chest pain; dyspnea; absent breath sounds; inaudible egophony, bronchophony, and whispered pectoriloquy; and increased resonance during percussion.

ALERT A pneumothorax that continues to increase in size may be life-threatening, particularly if the patient is being ventilated mechanically. If the increasing intrapleural air is not evacuated immediately, intrathoracic pressure may increase, causing decreased cardiac output, hypotension, and eventual death.

SOUND CHARACTERISTICS

Diminished or absent breath sounds resulting from a pneumothorax can be heard anywhere over the anterior, posterior, and lateral chest wall surfaces, depending on the location and size of the pneumothorax.

In a patient with a pneumothorax in the left lateral lung field — the area over the fourth, fifth, sixth, and seventh intercostal spaces between the anterior and posterior axillary folds — normal breath sounds are heard on the contralateral side over healthy lung tissue (♦30____), and breath sounds are absent over the pneumothorax. (♦31____) If diminished breath sounds are heard, they have a low pitch that is heard with either the bell or diaphragm of the stethoscope.

Pleural effusion

In pleural effusion, fluid accumulates in the pleural space, impairing the transmission of normal breath sounds. Because of the acoustical mismatch, breath sounds are diminished or absent. (♦32____)

A large pleural effusion compresses adjacent lung tissue, causing atelectasis; the percussion tone will be dull. Egophony, bronchophony, and whispered pectoriloquy caused by the atelectasis may be audible at the upper border of the pleural effusion. Occasionally, very loud bronchial breath sounds may have sufficient intensity to be transmitted through a small pleural effusion.

SOUND CHARACTERISTICS

Diminished or absent breath sounds resulting from a pleural effusion may be heard anywhere over the anterior, posterior, or lateral chest wall surfaces, depending on the location of the pleural effusion.

In a patient with a pleural effusion in the right posterior lower lung field, diminished breath sounds are heard over the eighth, ninth, and tenth intercostal spaces from the vertebral line to just right of the midscapular line (see *Pleural effusion affecting right lower lobe*), and normal breath sounds are heard on the contralateral side over healthy

Pleural effusion affecting right lower lobe

Affected lung area

Posterior auscultatory sites

lung tissue. (♦33____) The diminished breath sounds have a low pitch that can be heard with either the bell or diaphragm of the stethoscope. (♦34____)

ALERT If the pleural effusion is large, diminished or absent sounds will be heard over the lower right anterior and lateral chest wall surfaces as well. Monitor the patient for respiratory distress and prepare for chest tube insertion, if necessary.

Hyperinflated lungs

Hyperinflated lungs, typical of chronic obstructive pulmonary disease (COPD) or severe asthma, impede breath sound transmission in the following way: Premature dynamic compression of the large central airways and the loss of elastic tension in the lung tissue limit airflow during expiration. Increased intrinsic airway resistance may also be present. Increased amounts of air trapped in the lungs change the acoustical qualities of the sound transmitted, creating a mismatch between the pleurae and chest wall, and the hyperinflated lung tissue. (♦35____) Consequently, breath sounds are diminished.

The intensity of those breath sounds is directly related to the severity of the COPD. For example, patients with marked hyperinflation typically have an increased

Hyperinflated alveoli (hyperinflated lungs)

Auscultatory sites for COPD

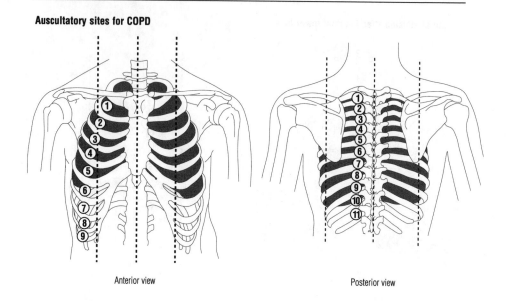

Anterior view

Posterior view

anterior-to-posterior thoracic diameter and a flattened and immobile diaphragm. Breath sounds are not as loud as usual because of the increased mismatch produced by trapped air and because less air is being moved during each respiratory cycle. Other signs and symptoms of COPD include a hyperresonant percussion note, dyspnea (a primary sign of severe COPD), and inaudible egophony, bronchophony, and whispered pectoriloquy.

ALERT Prepare for intubation and mechanical ventilation in a patient with COPD who has progressed from diminished to absent breath sounds.

SOUND CHARACTERISTICS
Diminished or absent breath sounds associated with COPD are heard over the anterior, posterior, and lateral chest wall surfaces. If the breath sounds are audible, they are soft in intensity and have a low pitch heard best with the diaphragm of the stethoscope. These sounds are heard throughout inspiration and expiration. (♦36____)

Obesity
Breath sounds are normally attenuated and filtered at the pleural surface. In an obese person, a thickened chest wall

increases the distance between lung tissue and the chest wall surface. This results in additional filtering of the breath sounds as they are transmitted from the pleurae to the chest wall surface. (♦37____)

Hyperinflated alveoli (PEEP)

Positive end-expiratory pressure
Adding PEEP during mechanical ventilation of an intubated patient can diminish breath sounds in the following way: PEEP increases functional residual capacity (FRC), the amount of air remaining in the airways at the end of normal expiration. Increasing FRC hyperinflates the lungs. Increased amounts of air in the small airways and alveoli change the acoustical qualities of the sound transmitted through the chest wall, creating a mismatch between the pleurae and chest wall, and the hyperinflated lung. Consequently, breath sounds are diminished. (♦38____)

◤ POSTTEST

1. What causes diminished or absent breath sounds?
2. Name six conditions associated with diminished or absent breath sounds.
3. Explain why shallow breathing results in diminished breath sounds.
4. Explain the effects of diaphragmatic paralysis on breathing.
5. Describe the changes in airflow distal to an obstruction.
6. Why does a pneumothorax cause diminished or absent breath sounds?
7. Describe the breath sound characteristics associated with a large pneumothorax.
8. What is a pleural effusion?
9. How does a large pleural effusion change breath sounds?
10. Describe the breath sound characteristics associated with a pleural effusion.
11. Why do hyperinflated lungs cause diminished or absent breath sounds?
12. Describe the breath sound characteristics associated with chronic obstructive pulmonary disease.

13. How does obesity change the characteristics of normal breath sounds?

14. Explain the effects of positive end-expiratory pressure on breath sounds.

Other Abnormal Breath Sounds

7

Classifying adventitious sounds

▶▌ *PRETEST*

1. Name two types of adventitious sounds.
2. Describe the difference between fine and coarse crackles.
3. Describe the difference between wheezes and low-pitched wheezes.

Confusion over terminology

Methods of classifying adventitious sounds have changed repeatedly over the years, resulting in continuing confusion in the literature and in the clinical setting. The familiar terms used by Laënnec were replaced by terms that later doctors thought were more aesthetic or clearer. For example, the term *rhonchus* was substituted for *rale* because the latter was associated with the death rattle sound. Later, attempts were made to classify adventitious sounds based on their acoustical qualities, or their similarities to musical tones.

Current classification system

In 1977, the American Thoracic Society adopted a system of classifying adventitious sounds based on acoustical qualities, timing, and frequency waveforms. This system divides adventitious sounds into two classifications: crackles and wheezes. These two classifications are further subdivided into two categories: discontinuous and continuous.

Discontinuous, explosive sounds that are loud and low-pitched are called *coarse crackles*. (♦39____) Previously, these sounds were called *rales* or *coarse rales*.

Discontinuous, explosive sounds that are shorter in duration, higher in pitch, and less intense than coarse crackles are called *fine crackles*. (♦40____) Previously, these sounds were called *fine rales* or *crepitations*.

Continuous sounds that are high-pitched and have a hissing or coughing sound are called *wheezes*. Wheezes often have a musical quality. (♦41____) Previously, these sounds were called *sibilant rales* or *sibilant rhonchi*.

Continuous sounds that are low-pitched and often resemble snoring are called *low-pitched wheezes*. (♦42____) Previously, these sounds were called *sonorous rales* or *sonorous rhonchi*.

◼◤ POSTTEST

1. Name the characteristics upon which the American Thoracic Society based its system of classifying adventitious sounds in 1977.
2. What are the two classifications of adventitious sounds?
3. Describe coarse crackles.
4. Describe fine crackles.
5. Describe wheezes.
6. Describe low-pitched wheezes.

8

Adventitious sounds: Crackles

▶️ PRETEST

1. What causes crackles?
2. Name the conditions associated with late inspiratory crackles.
3. Describe the characteristics of late inspiratory crackles.
4. What is the difference between coarse and fine crackles?
5. Name the conditions associated with early inspiratory and expiratory crackles.
6. Describe the characteristics of early inspiratory and expiratory crackles.
7. What are pleural crackles?
8. Describe the characteristics of pleural crackles.

Sound production

Crackles are short, explosive or popping sounds that are described according to their pitch, timing, and location. These characteristics change, depending on the underlying cause. Crackles are heard primarily through the chest wall with a stethoscope, but they may also be heard at the mouth with or without a stethoscope. Two different mechanisms are thought to generate crackles: air bubbling through secretions and the sudden explosive opening of airways.

Air bubbling through secretions

Air bubbling through secretions in the airways is widely accepted as one way crackles are produced. According to Forgacs, this explanation is probably true when the trachea and mainstem bronchi are full of sputum, as commonly occurs with severe pulmonary edema and chronic bronchitis. However, Forgacs argues that the air bubbling theory does not explain why crackles are heard mainly during inspiration and why they are heard over diseased lungs when sputum is usually absent. Further, in the smaller airways, airflow resistance, produced by the surface tension and viscosity of secretions, is too high to be overcome by the air pressure gradients that are present in healthy lungs during inspiration and expiration. Thus, another mechanism must explain how crackles are produced in the smaller airways.

Sudden explosive opening of airways

At the end of expiration, peripheral airways in the lung bases close. At the beginning of inspiration, these peripheral airways remain closed, and inspired air flows to each lung apex first. The airways that are distal to the closed peripheral airways remain underexpanded until airway pressures and external forces, such as diaphragmatic movement and rib cage expansion, snap the airways open. The sudden opening of multiple collapsed peripheral airways and the associated explosive changes in air pressures are thought to produce the crackles heard over the lung bases in a healthy person who inhales deeply after a maximum exhalation. This mechanism is also thought to be responsible for the crackles heard in patients with atelectasis and interstitial lung disease.

Crackles associated with the abrupt equalization of pressures and the sudden opening of peripheral airways are characterized by a repetitive rhythm and loudness. These characteristics suggest that the airways open in the same sequence, at the same point in the respiratory cycle, and at the same approximate lung volumes. Crackles may be present in the lung bases of elderly people and occasionally in other healthy individuals. These crackles clear with coughing and have no pathological significance.

Documentation

The timing of crackles is described as early, mid-, or late inspiration or expiration. Pitch is usually described as high or low. Intensity is variable and is described as loud or soft. Density is described as profuse or scanty. Duration, indicating the length of time that the crackles can be heard during inspiration or expiration, varies.

Late inspiratory crackles

Late inspiratory crackles are high-pitched, explosive sounds of variable intensity and density. They are heard most frequently over dependent or poorly ventilated lung regions.

Related conditions

Conditions associated with late inspiratory crackles include atelectasis, resolving lobar pneumonia, interstitial fibrosis, and left-sided heart failure.

Atelectasis

Atelectasis, incomplete expansion of a lung area, is seen in postoperative and immobile patients and in patients with impaired diaphragmatic function. This condition is caused by prolonged shallow breathing, by gravitational forces that close airways and deflate the lung bases, and by mucus plugging the airways. The result is poor ventilation in the affected areas and possible collapse of segmental or lobar bronchi. If small peripheral airways are involved, clinical findings may not be detectable. However, if a larger airway is involved, the clinical findings of decreased chest wall movement, a dull percussion note, and bronchial breath sounds are easily noted. Egophony, bronchophony, and whispered pectoriloquy typically are heard.

Crackles associated with atelectasis are produced by the sudden opening of collapsed small airways and adjoining alveoli. These crackles are high-pitched, explosive sounds heard late in inspiration. (♦43____)

SOUND CHARACTERISTICS

In a postoperative patient who has not been coughing and deep-breathing adequately, late inspiratory crackles are heard over the posterior bases of both lungs. (See *Late inspiratory crackles heard over lower lobes.*) This area is located between the eighth and tenth intercostal spaces from the left posterior axillary line to the right posterior axillary line. The crackles begin late in inspiration and become more profuse toward the end of inspiration. They vary in intensity but are high-pitched. (♦44____)

Because crackles associated with atelectasis are poorly transmitted to the chest wall surface, their intensity and density change when the stethoscope is moved only a short distance. They are not audible at the mouth. The

Late inspiratory crackles heard over lower lobes

Affected lung areas

Posterior auscultatory sites

patient's position also affects these crackles. For example, in an immobile patient, profuse crackles are heard in the dependent lung regions, but crackles are absent or scanty in nondependent lung regions. Also, crackles associated with atelectasis may clear somewhat with coughing.

Lobar pneumonia

In patients with resolving lobar pneumonia, crackles can be auscultated over lung areas where many alveoli are still filled with exudate, but the surrounding alveoli are aerated and have higher-than-normal ventilation. A large increase in air pressure gradients in the airways reaching these unaerated alveoli generates crackles as the airways are snapped open during late inspiration. These crackles have a sound similar to that of late inspiratory crackles heard over atelectatic areas, but they are not affected by coughing or position changes. (♦45____)

SOUND CHARACTERISTICS

In a patient with right middle lobe pneumonia, late inspiratory crackles are heard over the right anterior chest wall surface between the third and fifth intercostal spaces. They begin late in inspiration and become more profuse toward the end of inspiration. These crackles are typically high-pitched. (♦46____)

Late inspiratory crackles heard over right middle lobe

Affected lung area

Anterior auscultatory sites

Interstitial fibrosis

Diffuse interstitial fibrosis impairs or destroys alveoli by filling them with abnormal cells or by scarring the lung tissue. Unaffected alveoli are usually hyperaerated. The lungs become stiff and more difficult to inflate, and air-flow volumes usually decrease. Theoretically, the delayed opening of small airways during inspiration causes alveolar pressures in the affected lung tissue to fall more significantly than in healthy alveoli. This fall in alveolar pressures leads to an increased pressure gradient that generates repetitive late inspiratory crackles. (♦47____) Coughing does not affect the profusion of crackles.

In mild interstitial fibrosis, crackles are auscultated at the end of inspiration over dependent lung regions — usually over the lateral lung bases when the patient is seated upright. Crackles can disappear if the patient inhales deeply, holds his breath, or leans forward. However, they usually recur when the patient returns to the upright position.

As interstitial fibrosis worsens, crackles are heard bilaterally over the posterior lung bases and spread upward toward the apices. In later stages of the disease, crackles are not affected by position changes and may be heard throughout inspiration.

Either interstitial fibrosis or interstitial pneumonitis is associated with interstitial and alveolar infiltrates. Patients with a significant amount of lung involvement have

Lung areas where right and left lateral late inspiratory crackles are heard

Auscultatory sites for late inspiratory crackles heard over lateral lung bases

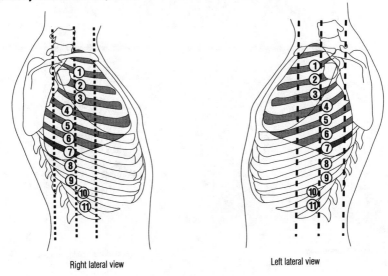

Right lateral view   Left lateral view

dyspnea and a cough. Interstitial fibrosis may be caused by inhalation of heavy metals, the antibiotic nitrofurantoin, some chemotherapeutic agents, or prolonged inhalation of high concentrations of oxygen. In most cases, however, the etiology is unknown.

Crackles heard in patients with known exposure to asbestos are thought to be an early sign of asbestosis, a lung disease characterized by pulmonary inflammation and fibrosis. The profusion of crackles increases in proportion to the amount of exposure to asbestos.

Pulmonary sarcoidosis, a noncaseating granulomatous disease of unknown etiology that occurs in the lungs and other organs, may progress to interstitial fibrosis, resulting in restrictive lung disease. The connective tissue disorders rheumatoid arthritis and scleroderma are also associated with diffuse interstitial fibrosis.

SOUND CHARACTERISTICS
Crackles associated with interstitial fibrosis caused by early asbestosis are initially heard in the midaxillary area over the lateral lung bases, the area over the seventh and eighth intercostal spaces. However, as the disease progresses, they may be heard over the posterior bases and may spread toward the apices. These crackles have a fine intensity and a short, discontinuous duration; they are heard dur-

Late inspiratory crackles heard over posterior lung bases

Affected lung areas

Posterior auscultatory sites

ing late inspiration. They have a high pitch heard best with the diaphragm of the stethoscope. (♦48____)

Left-sided heart failure

Left-sided heart failure leads to fluid accumulation in the lung interstitium. Crackles are produced by the rapid equalization of pressures associated with the delayed opening of airways narrowed by pulmonary edema. They're often auscultated over the posterior lung bases in the early stages of pulmonary edema. Profuse and high-pitched (♦49____), these crackles are inaudible at the mouth. Common symptoms of left-sided heart failure include rapid, shallow breathing and mild hypoxia. If pulmonary edema worsens, the airways are flooded with fluids. This results in severe hypoxia and low-pitched inspiratory and expiratory crackles that may be audible at the mouth and over the entire chest wall surface.

SOUND CHARACTERISTICS

Crackles associated with early left-sided heart failure and pulmonary edema are heard bilaterally over the posterior lung bases (see *Late inspiratory crackles heard over posterior lung bases*), the area over the eighth, ninth, and tenth intercostal spaces. However, as pulmonary edema worsens, the crackles become more profuse and may be heard throughout the chest during late inspiration. Their in-

Auscultatory sites for early inspiratory crackles

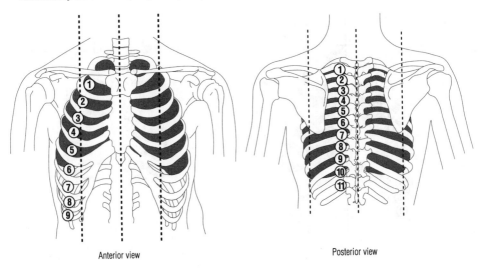

Anterior view

Posterior view

tensity is fine in the early stages of left-sided heart failure but changes to a loud rattling sound as the patient's condition worsens; duration varies with the degree of failure. The crackles have a low pitch that's heard best with either the bell or diaphragm of the stethoscope. (♦50____)

Early inspiratory and expiratory crackles

Coarse crackles occur during early inspiration and during expiration. They are common in diffuse airway obstruction and may be heard over any chest wall area. Coarse crackles have a lower pitch than fine crackles and, although they're usually loud, may disappear after a cough; they're unaffected by the patient's position.

Coarse crackles typically are heard in an irregular rhythm that may be interrupted by short sequences of evenly spaced crackles having the same intensity. They are thought to be produced by the intermittent closure of large bronchi and the corresponding flow of a bolus of air through the obstructed area.

Lung area where early inspiratory crackles are heard

Related conditions
These crackles are associated with chronic bronchitis and bronchiectasis.

Auscultatory sites for profuse early to midinspiratory crackles

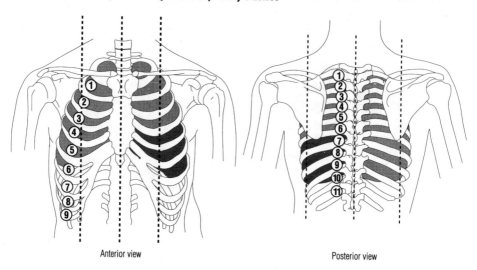

Anterior view

Posterior view

Lung area where profuse early to midinspiratory crackles are heard

Chronic bronchitis

Early inspiratory crackles are associated with excessive mucus production in patients with chronic bronchitis. The proliferation and hypertrophy of mucous glands within the airways are caused by chronic exposure to airway irritants, such as cigarette smoke (the most common) and air pollution. Cough, sputum production, and repeated respiratory infections are common in patients with chronic bronchitis. Chronic bronchitis can lead to chronic obstructive pulmonary disease. (♦51____)

SOUND CHARACTERISTICS

In patients with chronic bronchitis, crackles are heard early in inspiration, over all chest wall surfaces, and at the mouth. They are scanty and low-pitched and are not affected by the patient's position. (♦52____)

Bronchiectasis

Bronchiectasis, irreversible dilation of the bronchi in selected lung segments, is characterized by chronic and copious production of yellow or green sputum and by fibrotic or atelectatic lung tissue surrounding the affected airways. Evidence of old inflammatory changes in the patient's lungs is often noted on the chest X-ray.

The causes of bronchiectasis include foreign body obstruction, tumor, viral or bacterial pneumonia (particularly repeated childhood pneumonias), chronic inflammatory or fibrotic lung diseases, and tuberculosis. (♦53____)

Auscultatory sites for pleural crackles heard over right midlung

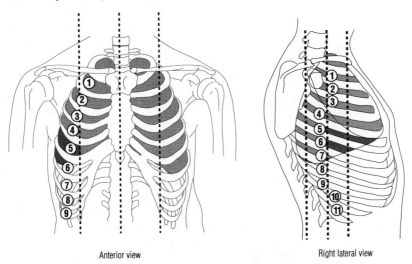

Anterior view   Right lateral view

SOUND CHARACTERISTICS

In patients with left midlung and lower lung area bronchiectasis, crackles are heard over the patient's anterior, posterior, and left lateral chest wall surfaces. The anterior area is located over the fourth, fifth, and sixth intercostal spaces, and the posterior area is located over the seventh, eighth, ninth, and tenth intercostal spaces. In patients with bronchiectasis, crackles tend to be profuse, low-pitched, heard during early or midinspiration, and coarser than those associated with chronic bronchitis. Coughing may decrease the number of crackles heard, but changes in the patient's position do not affect them. (♦54___)

Lung area where right midlung pleural crackles are heard

Pleural crackles

When the visceral and parietal pleural surfaces are damaged by fibrin deposits or inflammatory or neoplastic cells, they lose their ability to glide silently over each other during breathing, and their movements become jerky and periodically delayed. This motion produces loud, grating crackles known as *pleural crackles* or *pleural friction rub*. (♦55___) These crackles may be present during the inspiratory and expiratory phases of the respiratory cycle, or they may be confined only to inspiration. Pleural crackles disappear if fluid accumulates between the pleurae.

Pleural crackles are usually associated with sharp pain during inspiration, which may cause the patient to spontaneously splint the affected side to minimize muscle movement and chest expansion. Asymmetrical chest wall movement in the patient may be palpable, and a rapid, shallow breathing pattern may also be present.

SOUND CHARACTERISTICS

Pleural crackles are heard on the chest wall over the affected area. When pleural crackles are heard over the patient's right midlung — the area over the fifth and sixth intercostal spaces between the right midclavicular and right midaxillary lines — their intensity is loud and they have a coarse, grating quality and a low pitch. (♦56____) Their duration is discontinuous. Pleural crackles may be heard during inspiration only or during both the inspiratory and expiratory phases of the respiratory cycle.

AUSCULTATION TIP To distinguish between a pleural friction rub and a pericardial friction rub, have the patient hold his breath; if the rub continues, it's a pericardial friction rub.

POSTTEST

1. Define crackles.
2. Name two causes of crackles.
3. Explain how air bubbling through secretions produces crackles.
4. Explain how the sudden explosive opening of airways causes crackles.
5. What are the characteristics of crackles?
6. Name four conditions associated with late inspiratory crackles.
7. How does atelectasis generate crackles?
8. Describe the characteristics of crackles associated with atelectasis.
9. How are crackles generated in the patient with resolving lobar pneumonia?
10. Describe the characteristics of crackles associated with resolving lobar pneumonia.
11. How does interstitial fibrosis cause crackles?
12. What changes in crackles' characteristics would be expected as interstitial fibrosis worsens?
13. Describe the characteristics of crackles associated with interstitial fibrosis.

14. How are crackles generated in the patient with left-sided heart failure?
15. Describe the characteristics of crackles associated with left-sided heart failure.
16. How are coarse crackles thought to be produced?
17. Explain how early inspiratory crackles are generated in the patient with chronic bronchitis.
18. Describe the characteristics of crackles associated with chronic bronchitis.
19. What is bronchiectasis?
20. Describe the characteristics of crackles associated with bronchiectasis.
21. What causes pleural crackles?
22. Describe the characteristics of pleural crackles.

9

Adventitious sounds: Wheezes

▶❚❙ *PRETEST*

1. What causes wheezes?
2. What conditions are associated with wheezes?
3. Describe the following types of wheezes: expiratory polyphonic, fixed monophonic, sequential inspiratory, and random monophonic.
4. What type of wheeze is associated with asthma?
5. What type of wheeze is associated with widespread airflow obstruction?
6. What is stridor?

Sound production

Airflow pattern in narrowed bronchus

1. Airway wall
2. Narrowed bronchus

Airflow pattern in narrowed bronchus

1. Airway wall
2. Narrowed bronchus

Wheezes are musical sounds generated by air passing through a bronchus so narrowed as to be almost closed. The bronchus walls oscillate between closed and barely open positions; these oscillations generate audible sounds.

Wheezes are high-pitched, continuous sounds with frequencies of 200 Hz or greater and a duration of 250 msec or more. Their duration is long enough to carry an audible pitch similar to a musical tone. Wheezes are described by their timing within the respiratory cycle; they may be heard during inspiration, expiration, or continuously throughout the respiratory cycle. Wheezes can be further described as localized or diffuse, episodic or chronic.

A wheeze's pitch is determined by the emitted sound's frequency, which can vary widely over a five-octave range. These differences in frequency are attributed to the airway size and elasticity and to airflow rates through the narrowed bronchus. Theoretically, large, flabby, narrowed airways generate low-pitched sounds; stiff, narrowed airways generate high-pitched sounds. Pitch is not believed to be related to airway length or width or to air density.

Wheezes of different pitches may occur simultaneously or may overlap, and the pitch of a single wheeze may change during inspiration and expiration. *Monophonic wheezes* produce single musical notes that may vary in duration and may overlap. *Polyphonic wheezes* combine several distinct musical tones.

Wheezes are transmitted better through airways than through lung tissue, which absorbs high-frequency sounds. Wheezes that sound louder over central airways than over peripheral lung tissue may be sounds transmitted through the central airways but not produced by them. Wheezes heard at the mouth in severe airway obstruction may not be audible during auscultation of the chest wall surfaces.

ALERT Be alert for impending respiratory failure if wheezes are audible at the mouth and breath sounds are diminished or absent.

Conditions associated with wheezes include bronchospasm, airway thickening caused by mucosal swelling or muscle hypertrophy, inhalation of a foreign object, tumor, secretions, or dynamic airway compression.

Expiratory polyphonic wheezes

Polyphonic wheezes are believed to be caused by the dynamic compression of large airways during expiration. In healthy individuals, polyphonic wheezes can sometimes be auscultated during a maximal forced expiration when the dynamic compression occurs simultaneously in all airways. No regional variations exist in airway resistance or in lung compliance; consequently, polyphonic wheezes are heard throughout the lungs during expiration.

Polyphonic wheezes are loud and widely transmitted; when heard during regular breathing, they indicate widespread airflow obstruction.

In patients with widespread airflow obstruction (as in asthma and chronic bronchitis), elastic recoil properties, peripheral airway resistance, and airway mechanics are altered throughout both lungs. Together, these abnormal changes affect the timing of dynamic airway compression within the bronchi, which alters normal sound production. For example, during sequential forceful expirations, the central bronchi are compressed first when elastic re-

Auscultatory sites for expiratory polyphonic wheezes

Anterior view

Posterior view

Lung areas where expiratory polyphonic wheezes are heard

coil of the airways is low or when peripheral airway resistance is high. This compression produces a series of sounds, beginning with a monophonic wheeze and quickly followed by bitonal sounds. Very soon, the full complement of sounds that make up polyphonic wheezes are audible through the stethoscope. These multiple musical tones begin simultaneously and maintain a constant pitch that rises sharply at the end of expiration. (♦57____)

SOUND CHARACTERISTICS
Expiratory polyphonic wheezes are usually heard over the anterior, posterior, and lateral chest wall surfaces during expiration. Their intensity is usually described as loud and musical, and their duration is continuous. They have a high pitch heard best with the diaphragm of the stethoscope. (♦58____)

Fixed monophonic wheezes

Fixed monophonic wheezes, which have a constant pitch and a single musical tone, are generated by the oscillations of a large, partially obstructed bronchus. The obstruction may be caused by a tumor, a foreign body, bronchial stenosis, or an intrabronchial granuloma; each of these conditions narrows the airway but does not slow

Auscultatory sites for fixed monophonic wheezes

Anterior view

Posterior view

airflow. Fixed monophonic wheezes are low-pitched and are transmitted throughout the lungs. (♦59_____)

In a patient with bronchial stenosis, the pitch of inspiratory and expiratory monophonic wheezes varies, depending on airway rigidity. Monophonic wheezes may disappear when the patient is supine or turns from side to side.

Lung area where fixed monophonic wheezes are heard

Partially obstructed lobar bronchus

SOUND CHARACTERISTICS

In a patient with a partially obstructed right lobar bronchus, fixed monophonic wheezes are heard over the anterior, posterior, and right lateral chest wall surfaces. The anterior area is located over the third, fourth, fifth, and sixth intercostal spaces; the posterior area is located over the fifth, sixth, seventh, eighth, ninth, and tenth intercostal spaces. Fixed monophonic wheezes are usually loud, and their duration is continuous. They may be heard during inspiration, expiration, or throughout the respiratory cycle. They have a low pitch heard best with the diaphragm of the stethoscope. (♦60_____)

Sequential inspiratory wheezes

Sequential inspiratory wheezes are sometimes heard over the lung bases in patients with interstitial fibrosis, asbestosis, or fibrosing alveolitis. These monophonic wheezes

Lung areas where sequential inspiratory wheezes are heard

Auscultatory sites for sequential inspiratory wheezes

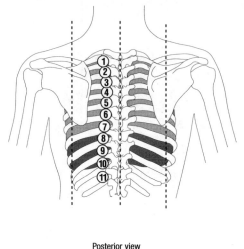

Posterior view

are generated by airways that open late in inspiration in unaerated lung regions. The rapid inflow of air precipitates airway wall vibrations, generating sequential inspiratory wheezes. A single, short inspiratory wheeze or a brief sequence of monophonic inspiratory wheezes with different pitches may be heard along with the crackles normally associated with interstitial fibrosis. (♦61____)

SOUND CHARACTERISTICS
Sequential inspiratory wheezes are usually heard over the lateral and posterior lung bases. On the posterior chest wall surface, this area is located over the eighth, ninth, and tenth intercostal spaces; on the lateral chest wall surfaces, it is located over the seventh and eighth intercostal spaces. Sequential inspiratory wheezes have a loud intensity and a continuous duration. They occur throughout inspiration but are more predominant in late inspiration. They have a high pitch heard best with the diaphragm of the stethoscope. (♦62____)

Random monophonic wheezes

Airways narrowed by bronchospasm or mucosal swelling produce single or multiple monophonic wheezes that may occur during inspiration, expiration, or throughout the res-

Auscultatory sites for sequential inspiratory wheezes

Right lateral view

Left lateral view

piratory cycle. Multiple wheezes can occur randomly and vary in duration. Random monophonic wheezes produced in the large central airways are loud and widely transmitted throughout the lung (see *Lung area where random monophonic wheezes are heard,* page 74); they can be heard at a distance from the mouth. (♦63_____) In contrast, random monophonic wheezes produced in the peripheral airways are weaker and are filtered as they are transmitted to the chest wall; these sounds are audible only over the chest wall.

Random monophonic wheezes are typically heard in patients with severe status asthmaticus. In such patients, airway resistance is high; dynamic airway compression moves from the central airways toward the smaller peripheral airways, where the airflow rate is too low to produce airway wall vibrations or sounds.

The progressive airway obstruction that occurs in patients with status asthmaticus can cause a dynamic pattern of wheezing. First, monophonic wheezes are heard only during expiration; then they are heard throughout the respiratory cycle. Monophonic wheezes may also be heard at the mouth because the high-frequency sounds are transmitted through larger airways.

ALERT As status asthmaticus becomes more severe, all wheezes heard over the chest wall surfaces disappear because a combination of air trapping

Lung areas where random monophonic wheezes are heard

Central airway spasm

and severe airway narrowing causes the site of dynamic airway compression to move toward the lung periphery; this phenomenon is called a silent chest. Silent chest is commonly accompanied by hypercapnia (increased carbon dioxide levels in the blood) and acidosis, both of which are life-threatening.

SOUND CHARACTERISTICS

Random monophonic wheezes are usually heard over the anterior, posterior, and lateral chest wall surfaces. They are usually loud, and their duration is continuous. These wheezes occur throughout the respiratory cycle, and expiration is frequently prolonged. They have a high pitch heard best with the diaphragm of the stethoscope. (♦64____)

Stridor

Stridor is a very loud musical sound that is heard at a distance from the patient, usually without a stethoscope. It is caused by laryngeal spasm and mucosal swelling, which contract the vocal cords and narrow the airway. The loud monophonic wheeze of stridor is typically heard during inspiration, but it also may be heard throughout the respiratory cycle as airway constriction increases. Its intensity distinguishes it from other monophonic wheezes. (♦65____) Stridor is associated with whooping cough, la-

Auscultatory sites for random monophonic wheezes

Anterior view   Posterior view

ryngeal tumors, tracheal stenosis, aspiration of a foreign object and, most commonly, severe upper respiratory infections.

SOUND CHARACTERISTICS
Severe stridor is heard without a stethoscope; however, in a patient with a less-pronounced laryngeal spasm, stridor may be heard by auscultating over the larynx. Stridor is very loud and has a continuous duration. It may be heard during inspiration or throughout the respiratory cycle. Its high pitch resembles a crowing sound. (♦66____)

ALERT If the patient with stridor is drooling, the epiglottis may be severely swollen. Don't examine the mouth. Any stimulus could worsen the airway occlusion. Immediate medical intervention is necessary. The patient may require intubation or emergency tracheotomy.

◢ POSTTEST
1. Define wheezes.
2. What are the characteristics of wheezes?
3. How is a wheeze's pitch determined?
4. How are wheezes transmitted?
5. Name five conditions associated with wheezes.
6. How are expiratory polyphonic wheezes generated?

7. How does widespread airflow obstruction change the sounds heard during auscultation?
8. Describe the characteristics of expiratory polyphonic wheezes.
9. How are fixed monophonic wheezes generated?
10. Describe the characteristics of fixed monophonic wheezes.
11. What conditions are associated with sequential inspiratory wheezes?
12. How are sequential inspiratory wheezes generated?
13. Describe the characteristics of sequential inspiratory wheezes.
14. How are random monophonic wheezes generated?
15. What condition is associated with random monophonic wheezes?
16. How can the characteristics of random monophonic wheezes be expected to change as asthma worsens?
17. Describe the characteristics of random monophonic wheezes.
18. What is stridor?
19. What causes stridor?
20. Describe stridor's characteristics.

SECTION **V**

Heart Sound
Fundamentals

10

The heart and auscultation

▶❚ *PRETEST*

1. Where is the heart located in the chest, and what are its dimensions in the average adult?
2. List the heart's chambers.
3. Name the atrioventricular and semilunar heart valves.
4. Describe the path of blood flow through the heart.
5. What are systole and diastole?
6. How do electrical impulses stimulate the heart muscle to contract?
7. Describe the path of the heart's conduction system.
8. Name the precordial sites recommended for auscultation of heart sounds.
9. What qualities should you look for in choosing a stethoscope?
10. What sound frequency is transmitted best by the bell of the stethoscope? By the diaphragm of the stethoscope?
11. What should you do to improve your ability to hear heart sounds more clearly during auscultation?
12. What are some maneuvers to enhance heart sounds during auscultation?

Anatomy and physiology

Heart location and size

The heart is a powerful muscle. Its primary functions are to pump deoxygenated blood to the lungs, where carbon dioxide-oxygen (CO_2–O_2) exchange takes place, and to pump oxygenated blood throughout the body. The top, or superior, part of the heart is called the base; the most inferior and lateral part of the heart is called the apex. The average-sized adult heart is approximately 4¾" (12 cm)

Dimensions of average-sized adult heart

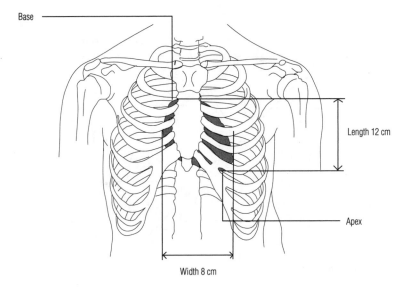

Base

Length 12 cm

Apex

Width 8 cm

long from the base to the apex and approximately 3⅛″ (8 cm) wide at its widest point. The heart gradually increases in size from infancy through early adulthood and usually is slightly larger in men than in women.

Right and left sides

Anatomically, the heart is divided into two functional sides: the right side and the left side, which are separated by the septum. Each side is further divided into chambers. The right atrium and right ventricle are the right-sided chambers; the left atrium and left ventricle are the left-sided chambers. (See *Right and left sides of heart,* page 80.)

Each chamber has unidirectional valves that separate the chambers and control blood flow. The right atrioventricular, or tricuspid, valve separates the right atrium and right ventricle, and the left atrioventricular, or mitral, valve separates the left atrium and left ventricle. The semilunar pulmonic valve separates the right ventricle and pulmonary artery, and the semilunar aortic valve separates the left ventricle and aorta. (See *Unidirectional heart valves,* page 80.)

Blood flow

Deoxygenated, or venous, blood from nearly every tissue of the body flows into the right atrium via the superior and inferior venae cavae. Venous blood from the heart tis-

Right and left sides of heart

Unidirectional heart valves

Pathway of deoxygenated blood through right heart to lungs

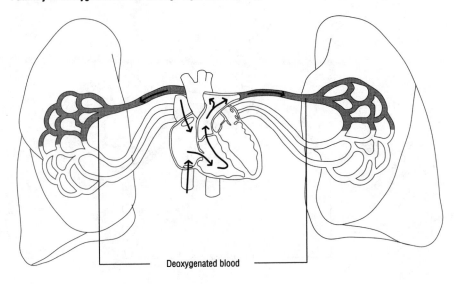

Deoxygenated blood

sue itself drains via the coronary sinus directly into the right atrium. The deoxygenated blood collects there until the tricuspid valve opens, and then it flows into the right ventricle. From the ventricle, it flows through the open pulmonic valve into the pulmonary artery, which distributes the deoxygenated blood to both lungs.

The complex process of CO_2–O_2 exchange occurs in the alveoli. Then the oxygenated blood flows back to the heart via the pulmonary veins and collects in the left atrium. From there, it flows through the opened mitral valve into the left ventricle. When the aortic valve opens, the oxygenated blood flows into the aorta, which transports it to all body tissues. (See *Pathway of oxygenated blood from lungs through left heart,* page 82.)

Heart as a pump

A healthy heart in a 154-lb (70-kg) adult pumps approximately 1⅝ gal (6 L) of blood per minute. Because the total blood volume in a healthy adult is about 1⅜ gal (5.2 L), the heart pumps the body's total blood volume in less than a minute. It performs this task continuously throughout an individual's life.

The flow of deoxygenated and oxygenated blood through the heart, lungs, and rest of the body is not a passive process. The heart must generate enough pressure to pump blood

Pathway of oxygenated blood from lungs through left heart

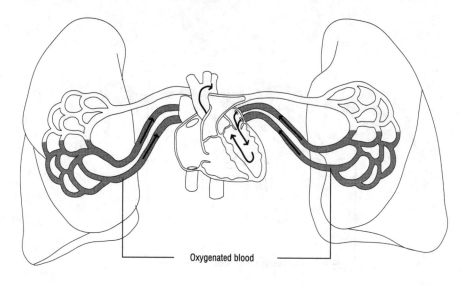

Oxygenated blood

through the arterial circulation. It does this by rhythmically contracting (systole) and relaxing (diastole).

During systole, heart muscle contraction raises the intracardiac pressures enough to systematically open the valves and pump a certain volume of blood. During diastole, the heart muscle relaxes, allowing the chambers to fill with blood again. This entire sequence is called the cardiac cycle.

The amount of blood pumped into the aorta each minute (cardiac output) is highly dependent on stroke volume. Stroke volume is the amount of blood pumped during each ventricular contraction.

Conduction system

Electrical impulses are primarily responsible for the heart's rhythmic pumping action. These impulses are discharged automatically from specialized cardiac cells that stimulate the heart muscle to contract. The specialized cardiac cells and fibers within the conduction system work together to produce a contraction. The impulses fired from the sinoatrial (SA) node, located just below the entrance of the superior vena cava in the right atrium, normally initiate the cardiac cycle, and they usually travel along specific pathways. For example, when the electrical impulse leaves the

Heart's conduction system

SA node
AV node
Bundle of His
Bundle branches
Purkinje fibers

SA node, it travels along the atrial conduction pathways located in the atrial walls, initiating atrial systole (or atrial contraction). The impulse very rapidly reaches the atrioventricular (AV) node, located near the atrioventricular junction. From the AV node, the impulse travels to the bundle of His located in the interventricular septum. Here the bundle of His divides into the right and left bundle branches. These branches further divide into the tiny Purkinje fibers located throughout the ventricular walls. As the impulse travels through the bundle branches and Purkinje fibers, it initiates ventricular systole (or ventricular contraction).

Cardiac cycle

Several mechanical events occurring simultaneously during the cardiac cycle enable the heart to pump oxygenated blood throughout the body.

During atrial diastole, when the right atrium and left atrium are relaxed, blood flows into the atria. The SA node, the pacemaker in a normally functioning heart, initiates an electrical impulse. The impulse is conducted via internodal pathways to both atria and results in atrial contraction. The open tricuspid and mitral valves allow blood to flow rapidly into the relaxed ventricles. The impulse is slowly conducted through the AV node, which allows time for the atria to contract completely and fill the ventricles with blood. From the AV node, the impulse is rapidly conducted through the bundle of His and its branches. The Purkinje fibers receive the impulse and directly stimulate the ventricular myocardium. The pulmonic and aortic valves open, and a forceful contraction of both ventricles ejects blood into the pulmonary artery and aorta.

The sequential and synchronized contraction (systole) and relaxation (diastole) of the atria and ventricles, along with the opening and closing of competent, properly functioning valves, ensure a unidirectional flow of blood through the heart and allow the heart to effectively move blood to all areas of the body quickly and repeatedly. However, this is not a silent process.

Traditional auscultatory areas

The heart's base normally lies beneath the sternum at the third intercostal space. Its apex is usually located between the fourth and sixth intercostal spaces, near or medial to the left midclavicular line. The apex is where apical pulses are taken and is usually the point of maximum impulse (PMI), the site where the heartbeat is seen or felt most strongly. But to auscultate for heart sounds and murmurs, specific precordial sites are used. These sites are the aortic, pulmonic, tricuspid, and mitral areas and Erb's point. Each area is named after the heart valve primarily responsible for the sounds that are heard best in that location.

The aortic area is located at the second right intercostal space close to the sternal border. Abbreviated as 2RSR, this area is where sounds of the aortic valve and aorta are heard best.

The pulmonic area is located at the second left intercostal space close to the sternal border. Abbreviated as 2LSB, this area is where the pulmonic valve and pulmonary artery sounds are heard best.

The tricuspid area is located at the fifth left intercostal space close to the sternal border. This area, abbreviated as 5LSB, is where sounds of the tricuspid valve and right ventricle are heard best.

The mitral area is located at or near the fifth intercostal space just medial to the left midclavicular line. This area, directly over the left ventricle, is sometimes referred to as the apical area, or apex. The mitral area, abbreviat-

Auscultatory areas

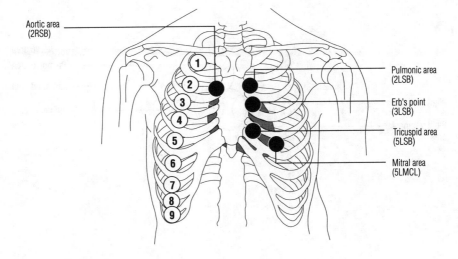

Aortic area
(2RSB)

Pulmonic area
(2LSB)

Erb's point
(3LSB)

Tricuspid area
(5LSB)

Mitral area
(5LMCL)

ed as 5LMCL, is where sounds associated with the mitral valve and left ventricle are heard best.

Erb's point differs from the four other areas in that it's not named after a heart valve, but it's a good location to hear sounds of aortic and pulmonic origin. Abbreviated as 3LSB, this area is located at the third left intercostal space close to the sternal border.

Alternative auscultatory areas

Although the traditional areas are a good reference for auscultating for heart sounds, it's important to know that the areas described can overlap extensively. Sounds produced by the heart's valves can be heard throughout the pericardium. Therefore, alternative auscultatory areas should also be considered when listening to the heart. (See *Alternative auscultatory areas,* page 86.)

The left ventricular area is located from the second to fifth intercostal spaces and extends from the left sternal border to the left midclavicular line. When the left ventricle is enlarged, this area extends in all directions. When the right ventricle is enlarged, this area is displaced to the left. The aortic component of the second heart sound A_2 and a left ventricular S_3 and S_4 are heard here. The murmurs of mitral or aortic stenosis and mitral or aortic insufficiency, a functional middiastolic rumble, and the mur-

Alternative auscultatory areas

murs associated with hypertrophic cardiomyopathy (formerly known as idiopathic hypertrophic subaortic stenosis) are best heard here.

The right ventricular area is located from the second to fifth intercostal spaces centered over the sternum. In severe right ventricular enlargement, this area may extend as far lateral as the point of maximum impulse. A right ventricular S_3 or S_4 and the opening snap of the tricuspid valve are heard here. Murmurs of tricuspid stenosis or regurgitation and ventricular septal defect are heard here.

The left atrial area is located from the second to fourth intercostal space at the left sternal border. The murmur of mitral regurgitation is best heard here.

The right atrial area is located from the third to fifth intercostal spaces at the right sternal border and may extend to or beyond the right midclavicular line in severe right atrial enlargement. This area is where the murmur of tricuspid insufficiency is heard best.

The aortic area is located from the right second intercostal space to the apex of the heart. The aortic ejection click and the aortic component of the second heart sound A_2 are heard best in this area. Murmurs of aortic stenosis and insufficiency, increased aortic flow, dilation of the ascending aorta, and abnormalities of the carotid and subclavian arteries are also heard here.

The pulmonic area is located at the second and third intercostal spaces close to the sternum but may be higher or lower. The pulmonary component of the second heart sound P_2 and the pulmonary ejection sound are heard here as well as the murmurs of pulmonary stenosis and insufficiency, increased pulmonary flow, patent ductus arteriosus, and stenosis of the main branch of the pulmonary artery.

Auscultatory techniques

The stethoscope

The stethoscope allows you to hear heart vibrations that are transmitted to the chest wall. These vibrations have various characteristics: Some are easily heard; others are less distinct. Consequently, the better the stethoscope, the better your chances of hearing subtle differences in the sounds.

Choose your stethoscope carefully. The chest piece should have a diaphragm and a bell. The diaphragm is designed to transmit high-pitched sounds more clearly, and the bell is designed to transmit low-pitched sounds more clearly. A flat, adult-sized diaphragm should be approximately $1^3/8$" (3.5 cm) in diameter and should be smooth, thin, and stiff enough to filter out low-frequency sounds. The bell should be approximately 1" (2.5 cm) in diameter and deep enough so that it does not fill with tissue when placed on the chest wall. The tubing length can vary from 10" to 15" (25 to 38 cm), and its inside diameter should be $1/8$" — or $3/16$" if the tubing is longer. The earpieces should fit inside the ears comfortably (covering the external ear canal), and the stethoscope should not be too heavy because its weight can interfere with your ability to hear sounds accurately.

Using the stethoscope

The way you use the stethoscope's diaphragm and bell affects the quality of the heart sounds and murmurs you hear during auscultation. To maximize the effectiveness of auscultation, you must hold the diaphragm and bell correctly.

To use the diaphragm, firmly grasp the metal area between the bell and the diaphragm with your finger and thumb, and press down firmly on the chest wall. Or place your fingertips on the bell's rim, and press down firmly against the chest wall. Apply enough pressure so that an indentation remains on the skin after you remove the stethoscope.

The bell, however, should touch the chest wall only lightly. If you exert too much pressure when listening with the bell, the stretched skin beneath it will act as a diaphragm, filtering out low-pitched sounds. To hold the bell correctly, grasp the diaphragm's outer edges with the index finger and thumb, and gently rest the bell on the chest wall. Look at the skin around the edges of the bell to see if too much pressure is being applied. If any signs of indentation appear on the skin, relax the downward pressure.

Also, remember to hold the chest piece so that the tubing is not touching the patient or you; such contact creates sounds that interfere with effective listening.

Auscultatory sequence

During auscultation, listen over all five auscultatory areas, first with the diaphragm and then with the bell. Be sure to listen through several cardiac cycles to allow yourself enough time to become oriented to the sounds and to hear any subtle changes. Try to establish a pattern, and follow it methodically each time you perform auscultation.

Before starting auscultation, place the patient in a supine position. You may elevate the head of the bed slightly if it is more comfortable for the patient. Then stand to

Auscultatory sequence

Aortic area

Pulmonic area

Erb's point

Tricuspid area

Mitral area

the patient's right. Listen first with the diaphragm over the aortic area. Try to recognize the characteristic lub-dub sound of each cardiac cycle. After listening through several cycles, inch the diaphragm toward the pulmonic area. Try to move the diaphragm without losing track of the lub-dub. Then listen over the pulmonic area, Erb's point, and the tricuspid area. Continue in this manner until you reach the mitral area.

To locate the PMI, turn the patient slightly to the left, placing him in the partial left lateral recumbent position. This position brings the heart's apex closer to the chest wall. Closely observe the chest wall for any sign of the heartbeat, which may appear as a rhythmic bulging. Then use your fingertip pads to palpate for the heartbeat between the fourth and sixth intercostal spaces, near the left midclavicular line. The chest wall site where the heartbeat is seen and felt is the PMI. In a healthy adult, the PMI and the mitral area are usually located at the same site.

After listening over the PMI with the diaphragm of the stethoscope, turn the chest piece so that you can use the bell. Then listen over the PMI with the bell. Reverse the auscultatory sequence, inching the bell over all the ausculatory areas.

If the patient can tolerate it, always auscultate for heart sounds in both supine and seated positions. Thus, after auscultating with both the bell and the diaphragm while the patient is in a supine position, have him sit up and lean forward slightly. Then repeat the entire auscultatory sequence with the diaphragm and the bell.

Enhancement techniques

Ensuring the proper environment

A quiet, comfortable environment is recommended during auscultation for heart sounds. Privacy and a warm room are beneficial because the patient's entire chest is exposed throughout the examination. Shivering or any muscular movement, for example, would interfere with heart sound transmission, making it impossible to accurately detect subtle characteristics of the sounds. Close the door and try to eliminate any mechanical noises in the room. If possible, also discontinue any I.V. pumps or oxygen delivery systems for a short time.

Some helpful maneuvers

Several maneuvers can enhance the heart sounds heard during auscultation. Besides the position changes described on pages 88 and 89, you can also use maneuvers that increase or decrease blood flow through the heart. For example, you can have the patient squat or stand, hold his breath, or raise his legs while in a supine position. Another common technique is to have the patient cough several times or perform Valsalva's maneuver. During this maneuver, the patient attempts to exhale forcefully against a closed glottis.

Another method that enhances the sounds heard during auscultation is to have the patient increase the depth of breathing. This decreases the respiratory rate and makes it easier to distinguish sounds originating in either the right or left side of the heart. For example, during inspiration, venous return is enhanced, accentuating right-sided cardiac events; during expiration, left-sided blood flow is enhanced, accentuating left-sided cardiac events.

You can help the patient by raising your hand slowly when you want him to inhale and then lowering your hand slowly when you want him to exhale. Caution the patient to breathe smoothly and continuously. Breath holding may produce a Valsalva-type maneuver, which will negate the cardiac responses being assessed.

K POSTTEST

1. What is the heart's primary function?
2. What are the base and apex of the heart?
3. How is the heart divided anatomically?
4. Name the four unidirectional valves.
5. Describe blood flow through the heart.
6. Give the approximate total blood volume of a healthy adult and the time it takes the heart to pump this total blood volume.
7. What happens in the heart during systole and diastole?
8. What are stroke volume and cardiac output?
9. Describe the conduction of electrical impulses in the heart.
10. Briefly describe the heart's pumping action.
11. What are the names and locations of the five auscultatory areas used during auscultation for heart sounds?

12. What characteristics should you look for when choosing a stethoscope?
13. Describe how to use the diaphragm and bell of the stethoscope correctly.
14. Describe the auscultatory sequence.
15. How do you locate the point of maximum impulse?
16. What can you do to enhance heart sounds?

11

Heart sound dynamics

▶❙❙ *PRETEST*

1. How do heart sounds originate?
2. Name the two basic heart sounds and the valves associated with each.
3. How many characteristics are used to describe heart sounds?
4. How does the electrocardiogram (ECG) correlate with the heart's electrical activity?
5. What is a phonocardiogram?
6. How can you accurately document the heart sounds heard during auscultation?

Heart sound origins

The heart sounds heard through a stethoscope during auscultation are generated by vibrations from the heart's walls and valves and from turbulent blood flow. Normally, the heart's walls and valves are compliant as they move in response to pressure and volume changes during the cardiac cycle.

Blood flow

At the beginning of ventricular diastole, the ventricles are relaxed, and the aortic valve closes slightly before the pulmonic valve. For a brief time, both the atrioventricular and semilunar valves are closed. During this period, called *isovolumic relaxation,* intraventricular pressures continue to fall. But the opening of the tricuspid and mitral valves follows quickly, and blood begins to flow passively from the atria into the ventricles. As the ventricles become distended, the rate of ventricular filling decreases. Then, as the atria contract (from stimulation of the atrial myocardium by an electrical impulse from the sinoatrial [SA] node), a slight boost in ventricular volume occurs. The resulting increase in ventricular pressures causes the mitral and tricuspid valves to begin closing.

During atrial systole, the electrical impulse moves more slowly through the atrioventricular (AV) node and into the bundle of His. The impulse proceeds rapidly through the bundle branches and the Purkinje fibers, activating ventricular systole. Early in ventricular systole, intraventricular pressures increase above intra-atrial pressures, and the mitral and tricuspid valves close suddenly. Normally, the mitral valve closes slightly before the tricuspid valve.

For another brief period, both the atrioventricular and semilunar valves are closed. During this period, known as *isovolumic contraction*, ventricular pressures increase, becoming higher than the pressures in the pulmonary artery and aorta. The aortic and pulmonic valves open, and blood is ejected through them. Normally, the aortic valve opens slightly before the pulmonic valve.

After a period of maximum ejection of blood from the ventricles, the ventricles begin to relax. As intraventricular pressures fall rapidly, a brief backflow of blood from the pulmonary artery and aorta toward the ventricles occurs. Reduced intraventricular pressures and the temporary backflow of blood are associated with closure of the aortic and pulmonic valves at the end of systole.

Basic heart sounds

A normally functioning heart produces two basic heart sounds: S_1 and S_2. (♦1____) S_1, the first heart sound, is heard at the beginning of systole. It's associated with closure of the mitral and tricuspid valves and the increasing pressures within the ventricles that cause the moving valve leaflets and cord structures to decelerate. (See *Valves producing first heart sound [S_1]*, page 94.) S_1 is generated by the closing of AV valves and the vibrations caused by tensing of the chordae tendineae.

At the end of ventricular systole, ventricular pressures fall rapidly, causing a slight backflow of blood from the aorta and pulmonary artery. The decrease in ventricular pressures to a level below that of aortic and pulmonic systolic pressures and the temporary backflow of blood and recoil events are associated with closure of the aortic and

Valves producing first heart sound (S₁)

Tricuspid valve (T₁)

Mitral valve (M₁)

pulmonic valves. The vibrations associated with these events produce the second heart sound, S₂, which marks the end of ventricular systole. (♦2____)

Characteristics

Every heart sound has six different characteristics that need to be assessed during auscultation. These are location, intensity, duration, pitch, quality, and timing. If you keep these characteristics in mind each time you perform auscultation, you will ensure a complete assessment of heart sounds, and you will be able to provide the information necessary for accurate and complete documentation. Also, because these terms are used universally, all health care professionals will be able to understand your auscultatory findings.

A sound's *location* is the anatomic area on the patient's chest wall where the sound is heard best. Bony structures and landmarks, such as the right and left midclavicular lines, are used to describe the precise location. For example, you might document that S₁ was heard best over the mitral area or at 5LMCL.

Intensity refers to the sound's loudness during auscultation. Usually, a sound's intensity is determined somewhat subjectively, based on experience. However, when

Valves producing second heart sound (S₂)

Aortic valve (A₂)

Pulmonic valve (P₂)

abnormalities are present, intensity can be determined electronically by recording a phonocardiogram (PCG) and by measuring the amplitude of the sound's vibrations. A PCG is a graphic representation of heart sounds that can be compared to the sounds heard during auscultation and to the heart's electrical activity recorded on the patient's electrocardiogram (ECG).

Keep in mind that heart sound intensity is related to the pressures generated and the blood flow velocity within the heart. It's also related to the patient's size, body build, and chest configuration. For example, a slender patient has a thinner chest wall; therefore, sounds are transmitted more easily through a slender patient's chest wall than through an obese patient's chest wall. Sounds can also be diminished by certain media, such as pericardial fluid or emphysematous lung tissue.

Sound *duration* refers to the length of time the sound is heard; it can be described as either short or long. Remember, heart sounds are brief vibrations that mark the beginning and end of systole. A sound's duration affects whether you hear it as a click, a snap, or a murmur. For example, murmurs are longer vibrations usually associated with blood flow during systole or diastole.

A sound's *pitch* is determined by the frequency of its vibrations. High-frequency sounds, like the notes of a piccolo, are best heard with the diaphragm of the stethoscope; low-frequency sounds, like the notes of a tuba, are best heard with the bell of the stethoscope.

Sound *quality* is determined by the combination of its frequencies. It may be described as sharp, dull, booming, snapping, blowing, harsh, or musical.

A sound's *timing* refers to when it's heard during the cardiac cycle — that is, during systole or diastole.

By using these six characteristics, you can describe precisely every heart sound, whether normal or abnormal. You can document what you heard, where you heard it, how you heard it, and when you heard it. Complete documentation also provides other health care professionals with invaluable information that helps them recognize subtle changes in the patient's heart sounds.

Depolarization and repolarization

The sequential and rhythmic process of depolarization and repolarization is referred to as the heart's electrical activity. Electrical activity occurs at the cellular level in every contractile cell of the myocardium.

Initially, the contractile cell is polarized (in a resting state). Depolarization begins when the cell membrane becomes permeable to the flow of sodium ions into the cell. Repolarization begins when calcium ions move into the cell and potassium ions begin to move out of the cell. Then, the accumulated intracellular sodium and calcium ions are extruded while the lost potassium is restored to the cell by the sodium-potassium pump, completing repolarization. The cell is polarized to its original ionic state, and the myocardium relaxes.

The ECG

Heart sounds are produced by mechanical events that occur in response to an electrical impulse originating in the SA node. This electrical impulse travels through the myocardium, activating the atria and ventricles. The ECG documents the timing and amplitude of the heart's electrical activity but does not reflect mechanical events in the heart.

The ECG correlates with the heart's electrical activity in the following manner. The SA node fires, triggering an atrial contraction. The P wave, part of the ECG wave

The ECG

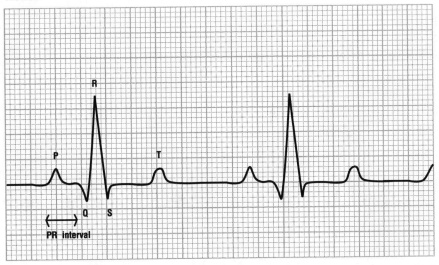

form, represents atrial depolarization. The QRS complex represents electrical depolarization of the ventricles. Atrial repolarization isn't seen in the ECG because it's hidden in the PR segment and the QRS complex. The T wave represents ventricular repolarization.

The impulse travels through the AV node, the bundle of His, the bundle branches, and the Purkinje fibers before the ventricles contract. The time between atrial contraction and ventricular contraction is recorded in the ECG as the PR interval: It begins at the onset of the P wave and lasts until the onset of the QRS complex.

ECG's relationship to first and second heart sounds

The first and second heart sounds directly correlate with a patient's ECG. S_1 normally occurs just after the QRS complex, and S_2 occurs at the end of the T wave. (See *Correlation of S_1 and S_2 with ECG*, page 98.)

Documenting heart sounds

The characteristics of each heart sound must be thoroughly documented. A phonocardiogram (PCG) provides one method of graphically representing heart sounds. (See *PCG and ECG showing S_1 and S_2*, page 98.) However, it isn't used

Correlation of S_1 and S_2 with ECG

PCG and ECG showing S_1 and S_2

Graphically documenting S$_1$ and S$_2$

routinely for every patient; therefore, a more practical graphic method of documenting heart sounds is recommended.

The intensity, duration, and timing of heart sounds can be represented graphically as rectangular blocks placed perpendicularly on a horizontal baseline. The block's height corresponds to the heart sound's intensity (the higher the intensity, the higher the block); the block's width corresponds to the sound's duration.

The proximity of one block on the baseline to the next block represents the time interval between one sound and another. The spacing between the blocks can also be used to specify the relationship of a particular heart sound to systole or diastole.

POSTTEST

1. How are heart sounds generated?
2. Describe what happens in the heart from the beginning of ventricular diastole to the beginning of atrial systole.
3. Describe what happens in the heart from the beginning of atrial systole to the beginning of ventricular systole.
4. Describe what happens in the heart from the beginning of ventricular systole to the beginning of ventricular diastole.
5. How is S$_1$ generated?
6. How is S$_2$ generated?
7. What is a heart sound's location?
8. What is a heart sound's intensity?
9. What is a heart sound's duration?
10. What is a heart sound's pitch?

11. What is a heart sound's quality?
12. What is a heart sound's timing?
13. Briefly explain the process of depolarization and repolarization.
14. Describe how the ECG correlates with the heart's electrical activity.
15. When do S_1 and S_2 occur in relation to the ECG waveform?
16. Describe a graphic method used to document heart sounds.

Normal Heart Sounds

12

The first heart sound

PRETEST

1. What is S_1?
2. What are the two basic components of the first heart sound?
3. Where is S_1 heard best?
4. Describe S_1, using six characteristics.
5. What is a widened S_1 split?

Normal S_1

The vibrations associated with closure of the mitral and tricuspid valves produce the first heart sound, S_1. Normally, only two components of the first heart sound are audible. The first component, referred to as M_1, is associated with closure of the mitral valve; the second component, T_1, is associated with closure of the tricuspid valve. Both valves close at the beginning of ventricular systole, but the mitral valve usually closes slightly ahead of the tricuspid valve.

Auscultatory area and relationship to ECG

M_1 and T_1 are usually perceived as a single sound called S_1, which is heard best near the heart's apex over the mitral area, using the diaphragm of the stethoscope. A single sound is heard because left heart sounds are normally more intense at this site. S_1 occurs just after the QRS complex in the electrocardiogram (ECG) waveform. ($\blacklozenge$3____)

As you inch the stethoscope from the mitral area toward the tricuspid area, without losing track of S_1, the M_1

Valves involved in S_1 sound production

1. Mitral valve
2. Tricuspid valve

PCG and ECG showing S₁

and T_1 components of S_1 become evident. Expiration makes them easier to hear. (♦4_____) T_1 trails M_1 slightly and is softer; it is heard best near the left sternal border. The timing of M_1 and T_1 with the QRS complex remains the same. (See *PCG and ECG showing normal S₁ split,* page 104.)

AUSCULTATION TIP If S_1 is difficult to identify, palpate for the carotid pulse while performing auscultation. S_1 will occur just before you feel the carotid pulse.

Auscultatory area for S₁

Mitral area

SOUND CHARACTERISTICS

S_1 is usually heard best near the heart's apex over the mitral area. Its intensity directly relates to the force of ventricular contraction and the amount of ventricular pressure developed during systole. S_1 is short in duration. You can hear its high pitch best with the diaphragm of the stethoscope. The quality of S_1 is somewhat dull. S_1 timing coincides with the beginning of ventricular systole and just precedes a palpable carotid pulse. (♦5_____) The characteristics of the normally split S_1 into M, and T, are the same. (♦6_____)

Auscultatory area for M₁ and T₁

1. Tricuspid area
2. Mitral area

ENHANCING S₁

S_1 can be enhanced by sympathetic stimulation such as that provided by a brief period of exercise.

PCG and ECG showing normal S₁ split

PCG and ECG showing abnormal S₁ split

Abnormal S₁ split

Widened S₁ split

The normal M_1-T_1 split heard over the tricuspid area widens when electrical activation and contraction of the right ventricle are delayed. Such a delay causes delayed tricuspid valve closure. (♦7____) This abnormal finding is associated with complete right bundle-branch block, left ventricular ectopic beats, epicardial pacing of the left ventricle, tricuspid stenosis, atrial septal defect, Ebstein's anomaly, and left ventricular tachycardia.

Auscultatory area for abnormal S₁ split

Tricuspid area

▌◀ POSTTEST

1. What produces the first heart sound, S_1?
2. What are the components of S_1?
3. Where is S_1 heard best during auscultation, and how does it change as the stethoscope is inched from one area to another?
4. Describe the characteristics of S_1.
5. How can S_1 be enhanced?
6. When does an abnormal S_1 split occur?
7. What conditions are associated with an abnormal S_1 split?

13

The second heart sound

▶‖ *PRETEST*

1. How does S_2 differ from S_1?
2. What are the components of S_2?
3. Describe S_2.
4. What is an S_2 split?
5. What types of S_2 splits may be heard during auscultation?

The vibrations associated with closure of the aortic and pulmonic valves produce the second heart sound, S_2. S_2 is usually louder than S_1 at the heart's base and usually slightly higher in pitch than S_1 at the heart's apex.

Normal S_2

S_2, like S_1, has two basic components: the aortic (A_2) component and the pulmonic (P_2) component. Both of these valves close at the end of ventricular systole. Normally, the aortic valve closes slightly ahead of the pulmonic valve.

Closing pressure is higher in the aorta than in the pulmonary artery; therefore, A_2 usually occurs earlier and is louder than P_2. (♦8____) Furthermore, A_2 can be heard over the entire precordium, whereas P_2 is usually auscultated over the pulmonic area.

Auscultatory area and relationship to ECG

To hear both components of S_2, listen carefully with the diaphragm of the stethoscope over the pulmonic area. Listen for S_2 just after the T wave in the patient's ECG.

Valves involved in S_2 sound production

1. Aortic valve
2. Pulmonic valve

PCG and ECG showing S₂

SOUND CHARACTERISTICS

S_2 is usually heard best near the heart's base over the pulmonic area or over Erb's point. Its intensity directly relates to the amount of closing pressure in the aorta and pulmonary artery. S_2 is slightly shorter in duration than S_1. You can hear its high pitch best with the diaphragm of the stethoscope. The quality of S_2 is somewhat booming; its timing coincides with the end of ventricular systole. (♦9_____)

Auscultatory area for S₂

1. Pulmonic area
2. Erb's point

S₂ split sounds

Normal S₂ split

The splitting of S_2 into the A_2 and P_2 components is heard best during inspiration over Erb's point. Remember, inspiration causes an increase in venous return to the right side of the heart. This increased venous return prolongs right ventricular ejection time, thus delaying P_2, or closure of the pulmonic valve. A decrease in blood flow to the left side of the heart occurs simultaneously, resulting in a shorter left ventricular ejection time.

Therefore, A_2 is heard earlier than P_2. (♦10_____) This means that a normal S_2 split is heard during inspiration, and the A_2 and P_2 components fuse during expiration.

Auscultatory area for normal S₂ split

Erb's point

PCG and ECG showing respiratory changes in normal S₂ split

While listening to S_2, you must determine the intensity of the A_2 and P_2 components and note the duration of the $A_2 - P_2$ interval as well as its relationship to the respiratory cycle. (♦11____) You should also document the S_2 split, noting whether the $A_2 - P_2$ interval increases or decreases during inspiration and expiration.

Changes in A₂ and P₂ intensity

The intensity of A_2 and P_2 changes proportionally with the difference in pressure gradients across the closed aortic and pulmonic valves. For example, P_2 may be louder than normal in conditions associated with elevated pulmonary artery diastolic pressure, as occurs in some patients with heart failure, mitral stenosis, Eisenmenger's syndrome, or other congenital heart diseases. When P_2 increases in intensity, it's sometimes heard over the mitral area and along the left sternal border. (♦12____)

A_2 intensity increases when diastolic pressure in the aorta increases. (♦13____) This commonly happens during exercise; during states of excitement such as extreme fear; in hyperkinetic conditions, such as thyrotoxicosis, fever, and pregnancy; and in systemic hypertension. However, if the patient has left ventricular decompensation, ventricular relaxation is slower, and the pressure gradients may not be great enough to produce an accentuated A_2.

PCG and ECG showing abnormal S₂ split with no respiratory variation

Conversely, A_2 intensity may be diminished in conditions that alter the development of diastolic pressure gradients, such as aortic regurgitation and hypotension. (♦14____) A_2 intensity also decreases when ventricular dysfunction is present, such as after an acute myocardial infarction. In this condition, P_2 may become louder if pulmonary artery pressure rises and systemic pressure falls.

Abnormal S₂ splits

Abnormal splitting is related to valvular dysfunction, to alterations in blood flow to or from the ventricles, or to both. These changes may cause the normal S_2 split to be absent during both phases of the respiratory cycle. Thus, only a single S_2 is heard over Erb's point. In another case, the split sounds may persist through inspiration and expiration with little or no respiratory variation. (♦15____) The split sounds may also be heard paradoxically on expiration. The $A_2 - P_2$ intervals vary, as does the intensity of A_2 and P_2 during the respiratory cycle. (♦16____) Changes in S_2 splits are usually most noticeable at the beginning of inspiration and expiration.

Absent S₂ split

The P_2 component may not be heard during auscultation over Erb's point in the patient with severe pulmonic steno-

PCG and ECG showing abnormal S₂ splits during respiratory cycle

sis. Consequently, S_2 remains a single sound during both inspiration and expiration. A normal S_2 split may also be absent if the A_2 sound masks the P_2 sound or vice versa — for example, when one sound is significantly louder than the other, making splitting inaudible. This phenomenon occurs in patients with pulmonary hypertension. On the other hand, systemic hypertension causes A_2 to be delayed and to fuse with P_2 during inspiration.

Persistent S₂ split

A persistent S_2 split occurs when A_2 and P_2 do not fuse into one sound during expiration, even though some respiratory variation in the intensity of A_2 and P_2 is heard. (♦17____) This persistent $A_2 - P_2$ splitting during expiration usually results from early aortic valve closure or delayed pulmonic valve closure.

Early aortic valve closure is associated with shortened left ventricular systole, which occurs in patients with mitral regurgitation, ventricular septal defects, or cardiac tamponade. Delayed pulmonic valve closure occurs when right ventricular systole is prolonged in patients with chronic pulmonary hypertension. In these patients, the $A_2 - P_2$ split is heard, but the interval between the A_2 and P_2 components is narrowed. (♦18____)

PCG and ECG showing persistent S₂ split

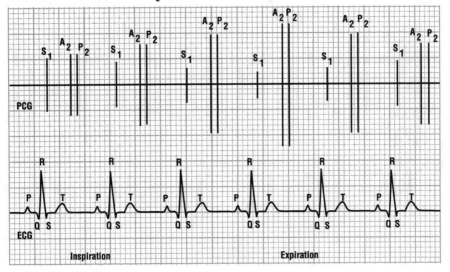

PCG and ECG showing narrowed S₂ split in a patient with chronic pulmonary hypertension

PCG and ECG showing wide, fixed S₂ split

Another cause of persistent $A_2 - P_2$ splitting throughout expiration is delayed electrical activation of the right ventricle, which will delay P_2. This phenomenon is commonly found in patients with right bundle-branch block, left ventricular epicardial pacing, or left ventricular ectopic beats.

Wide, fixed S₂ split

A prolonged right ventricular ejection time produces expiratory $A_2 - P_2$ splits that are widened and that persist even when the patient is seated. (♦19____) This occurs in patients with atrial septal defects, acute pulmonary hypertension secondary to massive pulmonary emboli, or pulmonic stenosis. The P_2 component may not be audible at all in patients with severe pulmonic stenosis.

A wide, fixed S_2 split is sometimes associated with the pulmonary vascular bed's increased capacitance (ability to receive blood volume and the decreased resistance that accompanies it). (♦20____) This phenomenon occurs in patients with idiopathic dilation of the pulmonary artery or with atrial septal defects. This split does not change with respiration.

Paradoxical S₂ split

In a paradoxical, or reversed, S_2 split, P_2 precedes A_2 and the split sounds are heard during expiration instead of inspiration. (♦21____) This phenomenon is almost always

PCG and ECG showing paradoxical S$_2$ split during expiration

caused by delayed aortic valve closure. If A$_2$ is delayed during expiration, it may follow P$_2$ causing an S$_2$ split; if A$_2$ is delayed during inspiration, A$_2$ and P$_2$ fuse because inspiration normally delays P$_2$. Therefore, S$_2$ is heard as a single sound during inspiration instead of a normally split sound. (♦22____)

Delayed A$_2$ is commonly seen in patients with delayed activation of the left ventricle caused by left bundle-branch block. It's also associated with right ventricular ectopic beats or right ventricular endocardial pacing. Prolonged left ventricular systole can also cause a delay in A$_2$. The same paradoxical P$_2$–A$_2$ split may be heard in patients with left ventricular failure, patent ductus arteriosus, coarctation of the aorta, tricuspid regurgitation, early right ventricular activation across accessory tracks as in Wolf-Parkinson-White syndrome, or ischemic heart disease.

Left ventricular pressure overload, which occurs in patients with systemic hypertension and hypertrophic cardiomyopathy, may also cause paradoxical S$_2$ split. Likewise, aortic stenosis may lead to paradoxical splitting of A$_2$ and P$_2$; however, if the stenosis is severe, the A$_2$ component may not be audible.

With left ventricular volume overload, which is commonly associated with aortic regurgitation or patent ductus arteriosus, A$_2$ may be delayed and a paradoxical S$_2$ split may be heard. But this isn't a common occurrence.

◪ POSTTEST

1. What produces the second heart sound, S_2?
2. What are the two basic components of S_2?
3. Where is S_2 heard best?
4. Describe the characteristics of S_2.
5. How does respiration affect S_2?
6. What clinical conditions change the intensity of A_2 and P_2?
7. Describe an abnormal S_2 split.
8. How do severe pulmonic stenosis and pulmonary hypertension affect the S_2 split?
9. Describe a persistent S_2 split.
10. Describe a wide, fixed S_2 split.
11. Describe a paradoxical S_2 split.

14

The third and fourth heart sounds

▶️ PRETEST

1. What are left ventricular diastolic filling sounds?
2. How do S_3 and S_4 differ from S_1 and S_2?
3. Describe a normal S_3.
4. Describe an abnormal S_3.
5. What is a right-sided S_3?
6. What is a ventricular gallop, or gallop rhythm?
7. What is an atrial diastolic gallop?
8. What is a pericardial knock?
9. Describe a normal S_4.
10. Describe an abnormal S_4, a summation gallop, and a right-sided S_4.

Ventricular filling sounds

The first and second heart sounds, S_1 and S_2, mark the beginning and end, respectively, of ventricular systole. In healthy individuals, these two sounds and their components are relatively easy to hear during auscultation and are best heard with the diaphragm of the stethoscope.

Two additional left ventricular diastolic filling sounds, S_3 and S_4, are sometimes heard over the mitral area. These sounds differ from S_1 and S_2 in that they are low-frequency sounds and are produced by ventricular filling rather than by valve closure.

Third heart sound

Normal S_3

Occasionally, a physiologic third heart sound, S_3, is heard during auscultation. This heart sound, considered normal

Area producing S₃

1. Mitral valve
2. Left ventricle
3. Tricuspid valve

Auscultatory area for S₃

Mitral area

in healthy individuals under age 40, is caused by vibrations occurring during rapid, passive ventricular filling. Early in diastole, after isovolumic relaxation, the mitral and tricuspid valves open and the ventricles fill and expand. In children and young adults, the left ventricle is normally compliant, permitting rapid filling. The left ventricle responds to this rapid filling with an abrupt change in wall motion that causes a sudden decrease in blood flow. These events generate vibrations that are responsible for the physiologic S_3. The more vigorously the left ventricle expands, the greater the likelihood that an S_3 will occur.

A physiologic S_3 is also commonly audible in patients with high-output conditions, in which rapid ventricular expansion, caused by increased blood volume, is present. Anemia, fever, pregnancy, and thyrotoxicosis are some of the conditions that cause rapid ventricular expansion, resulting in an S_3. An S_3 is also commonly heard in young, slender individuals during periods of excessive catecholamine release.

Auscultatory area and relationship to ECG

Usually, S_3 is heard best with the bell of the stethoscope over the mitral area, and it can often be palpated over the same area. It's heard best during expiration when blood flow into the left ventricle is increased. (♦23____) S_3 is heard early in diastole and follows S_2 by 0.14 to 0.20 second. The relationship of S_3 to the electrocardiogram (ECG) waveform can be seen easily on a phonocardiogram (PCG); in the ECG, S_3 occurs during the TP interval just after the T wave. Normally, the $S_2 - S_3$ interval is reliably constant.

SOUND CHARACTERISTICS

S_3 is usually heard best near the heart's apex over the mitral area. In some patients, it's soft and faint in intensity and difficult to hear; in others, it may be loud and easy to hear. S_3 has a short duration, and it may occur only intermittently during every third or fourth heartbeat.

S_3 has a low pitch that is heard best with the bell of the stethoscope, and it usually has a dull, thudlike quality. Its timing is closely related to S_2, which is heard just after the T wave; S_3 follows S_2 by less than 0.20 second. (♦24____)

ENHANCING S₃

Because S_3 is associated with blood volume and velocity, it can be intensified by maneuvers that increase stroke

PCG and ECG showing physiologic S$_3$

volume, such as elevating the patient's legs from a recumbent position or having the patient exercise briefly or cough several times. A physiologic S$_3$ often disappears with maneuvers that decrease venous return, such as having the patient sit up or stand.

AUSCULTATION TIP To enhance your ability to auscultate and palpate for an S$_3$, place the patient in a partial left lateral recumbent position.

Abnormal S$_3$

The left ventricle becomes less compliant with age. Decreased ventricular compliance leads to pressure changes, which cause slowed left ventricular isovolumic relaxation and reduced blood flow velocity into the ventricle. Thus, an audible S$_3$ after age 40 is considered abnormal. The S$_1$, S$_2$, S$_3$ sequence is referred to as a *ventricular gallop* or *gallop rhythm*. (♦25____) An abnormal S$_3$ has the same sound characteristics, is heard over the same location, and has the same timing in relation to S$_2$ as a physiologic S$_3$. The differences between the two are related to the patient's age, clinical condition, or both. Also, an S$_3$ gallop rhythm usually persists despite maneuvers that decrease venous return. (♦26____) (See *PCG and ECG showing abnormal* S$_3$, page 118.)

Area producing abnormal S$_3$

1. Mitral valve
2. Thickened left ventricle
3. Tricuspid valve

PCG and ECG showing abnormal S₃

PCG and ECG showing pericardial knock

An abnormal S_3 is almost always associated with increased mean left atrial pressure caused by a noncompliant left ventricle. This auscultatory finding is heard in patients with hypertrophic cardiomyopathy and frequently indicates elevated left ventricular diastolic pressure, as occurs in patients with heart failure.

An abnormal S_1 may also be heard in conditions associated with increased blood volume and increased inflow velocity into the left ventricle. It is heard with or without an increase in ventricular diastolic pressure. Consequently, patients with mitral regurgitation and constrictive pericarditis will have an abnormal S_3. This heart sound can also be heard during increased blood flow through the mitral valve, which occurs in patients with ventricular septal defects, patent ductus arteriosus, or severe aortic regurgitation.

An abnormal S_3 in patients with constrictive pericarditis is called a *pericardial knock*. This type of abnormal S_3 occurs closer to S_2. The interval between S_2 and S_3 is usually less than 0.14 second. (◆27____) The pericardial knock is easier to hear than a physiologic or abnormal S_3 and is heard best over the third, fourth, and fifth intercostal spaces along the left sternal border. (◆28____)

Right-sided S_3

Because the right ventricle is normally much more compliant than the left ventricle, its filling should not cause the vibrations that would create a right-sided S_3. However, in some patients, an S_3 originates in the right ventricle instead of the left. When it does, it's always considered abnormal. (◆29____) A right-sided S_3 is heard best over the third, fourth, and fifth intercostal spaces along the left sternal border and over the epigastric area. It's more prominent during inspiration because of increased blood flow into the right ventricle. (See *PCG and ECG showing right-sided S_3*, page 120.)

Patients with enlarged right ventricles and high right atrial pressures commonly have right-sided S_3. This heart sound is audible in patients with cor pulmonale secondary to pulmonary emboli or to parenchymal or vascular disease, right ventricular failure secondary to mitral stenosis with left-sided heart failure, pulmonary hypertension, ventricular septal defect, pulmonic regurgitation, or severe tricuspid insufficiency. (◆30____)

Auscultatory area for pericardial knock

1. Third intercostal space
2. Fourth intercostal space
3. Fifth intercostal space

Area producing right-sided S_3

1. Mitral valve
2. Tricuspid valve
3. Right ventricle

Auscultatory area for right-sided S_3

1. Third intercostal space
2. Fourth intercostal space
3. Fifth intercostal space
4. Epigastric area

PCG and ECG showing right-sided S₃

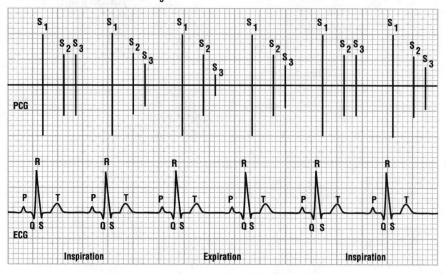

PCG and ECG showing S₄

Fourth heart sound

Normal S_4

By the end of diastole, the ventricles are nearly full; atrial contraction further stretches and fills the ventricles. The vibrations caused by this filling and stretching in late diastole generate an additional heart sound, S_4, sometimes called an *atrial diastolic gallop*. (♦31___) S_4 may be heard in patients of any age as well as in young athletes with physiologic left ventricular hypertrophy.

Because S_4 is associated with atrial contraction, it is not produced in conditions in which atrial systole does not occur, such as atrial fibrillation.

1. Mitral valve
2. Left ventricle

Auscultatory area and relationship to ECG

S_4 is usually heard best with the bell of the stethoscope during expiration near the heart's apex over the mitral area; it also may be palpable in this area. The relationship of S_4 to S_1 can be seen easily in the ECG waveform: S_4 occurs during the PR interval and precedes S_1.

Mitral area

SOUND CHARACTERISTICS

S_4 is usually located near the heart's apex over the mitral area; occasionally, it's also palpable over this area. In some patients it's faint in intensity and difficult to hear, but in others it's loud and easily heard. S_4 is relatively short in duration and may occur only intermittently, during every third or fourth heartbeat. It has a low pitch heard best with the bell of the stethoscope and a thudlike quality. Its timing is presystolic: S_4 precedes S_1 and occurs during the PR interval. (♦32___)

AUSCULTATION TIP To enhance S_4, place the patient in the partial left lateral recumbent position, which brings the heart closer to the chest wall.

Abnormal S_4

An abnormal S_4 is heard in numerous conditions, including hypertension (the most common cause), hypertrophic cardiomyopathy, cardiomyopathies, ischemic heart disease, and during or after an acute myocardial infarction. When an S_4 is heard in a patient with hypertension, the systolic blood pressure usually exceeds 160 mm Hg or the diastolic pressure exceeds 100 mm Hg.

Area producing right-sided S₄

1. Mitral valve
2. Tricuspid valve
3. Right ventricle

Auscultatory area for right-sided S₄

1. Third intercostal space
2. Fourth intercostal space
3. Fifth intercostal space
4. Epigastric area

An abnormal S_4 can also accompany volume overload conditions, such as hyperthyroidism, severe anemia, and sudden severe mitral regurgitation.

Summation gallop

Normally, S_4 precedes S_1 by an appreciable interval that correlates with the PR interval on the ECG. However, in patients with first-degree atrioventricular block, the P wave occurs early in diastole, and S_4 may occur during the early rapid diastolic filling period. Likewise, in tachycardia, S_4 may be superimposed on S_3 during early rapid filling. If either of these conditions exists, the S_4 fuses with S_3 to become a single diastolic filling sound called a *summation gallop,* which may be louder than S_4, S_3, or S_1. (♦33____)

Right-sided S_4

An S_4 generated in the right ventricle is called a *right-sided* S_4. (♦34____) It's commonly heard in conditions that increase pressure in the right ventricle by more than 100 mm Hg, such as pulmonic stenosis or pulmonary hypertension. This heart sound is heard best over the third, fourth, and fifth intercostal spaces along the left sternal border and over the epigastric area with the patient in a supine position; it's more audible during inspiration.

Differentiating S_4 from an S_1 split

Distinguishing an S_1 split $(M_1 - T_1)$ from an $S_4 - S_1$ sequence is sometimes difficult; however, here are some ways to help you do so. An S_1 split is heard best between the mitral and tricuspid areas with the diaphragm of the stethoscope, whereas an S_4 is heard best over the mitral area with the bell of the stethoscope and is usually not audible with the diaphragm. Also, an S_4 may be palpable and will disappear when the patient stands.

◎ **AUSCULTATION TIP** To increase the intensity of S_4, have the patient perform maneuvers that increase venous return to the heart, such as exercising briefly, squatting, or raising the legs while in a recumbent position.

PCG and ECG showing summation gallop

PCG and ECG showing right-sided S$_4$

S_3 and S_4: Similarities and differences

S_3, like S_4, is low-pitched and may be faint or loud and heard only intermittently. Both sounds are heard best over the mitral area, using the bell of the stethoscope, with the patient in a partial left lateral recumbent position. Both sounds are intensified by expiration and can be enhanced by maneuvers that increase stroke volume, such as elevating the legs while in a recumbent position.

The absence of S_3 and presence of S_4 indicate a compensated cardiac state. However, if the mean left atrial pressure rises, an abnormal S_1 may become audible. This is associated with a more serious prognosis for the patient.

█ POSTTEST

1. What are the two left ventricular diastolic filling sounds, and how do they differ from S_1 and S_2?
2. How is an S_3 produced?
3. List the conditions associated with an S_3.
4. Where and when is S_3 heard best?
5. Describe the characteristics of S_3.
6. What maneuvers can be used to enhance S_3?
7. An abnormal S_3 has the same sound characteristics, is heard at the same location, and has the same timing in relation to S_2 as a physiologic S_3. What is the difference between the two sounds?
8. What conditions are associated with an abnormal S_3?
9. Describe the characteristics of a right-sided S_3.
10. How is an S_4 produced?
11. Describe the characteristics of S_4.
12. How can an S_4 be enhanced?
13. In what conditions is an abnormal S_4 heard?
14. Describe a summation gallop.
15. Describe a right-sided S_4.
16. How can you differentiate between an S_4 and an S_1 split?
17. Compare and contrast S_3 and S_4.

Abnormal Heart Sounds

15

Other diastolic and systolic sounds

PRETEST
1. What causes an opening snap?
2. How can you differentiate an opening snap from S_2 and S_3?
3. What causes systolic ejection sounds?
4. What is the difference between a pulmonic ejection sound and an aortic ejection sound?
5. What is a midsystolic click (MSC)?
6. How can you differentiate an MSC from other heart sounds?

Opening snaps

At the end of ventricular systole, the aortic and pulmonic valves close, generating the second heart sound, S_2. S_2 is followed by a brief period of isovolumic relaxation; during this time ventricular pressures fall. When ventricular pressures are less than atrial pressures, the mitral and tricuspid valves open. Normally, the opening of these heart valves isn't audible. However, if the mitral valve leaflets become stenotic or abnormally narrowed while remaining somewhat mobile, they create an *opening snap* (OS). (♦35___) The OS sound is generated by the maximum, but limited, opening of the stenotic leaflets and usually indicates the beginning of the diastolic murmur associated with mitral stenosis. If the mitral valve becomes severely calcified and inflexible, the OS disappears.

Auscultatory area and relationship to ECG
An OS is heard best with the diaphragm of the stethoscope near the heart's apex over the mitral area or just medial to it. It's transmitted widely across the precordium

Area producing opening snap

Stenotic mitral valve leaflets

PCG and ECG showing opening snap

and can often be heard over the aortic, pulmonic, and tricuspid areas as well. An OS is higher in pitch than S_2; it may be as loud as or louder than S_2. An OS occurs early in ventricular diastole; thus, it's heard just after the T wave in the electrocardiogram (ECG) waveform.

SOUND CHARACTERISTICS

An OS is usually heard best near the heart's apex over the mitral area or just medial to it. Its intensity varies among patients, and it's usually easy to hear during auscultation. An OS has a short duration. It has a high pitch heard best with the diaphragm of the stethoscope and a sharp, snap-like quality. Its timing is closely related to S_2; an OS occurs early in ventricular diastole, just after the stenotic mitral valve opens. (♦36____)

Differentiating an OS from S_2

An OS occurs early in diastole and consequently may be confused with P_2 or S_3. One characteristic of an OS that helps distinguish it from P_2 is its timing: The $A_2 - P_2$ interval is normally shorter than the $A_2 - OS$ interval. Also, when the patient stands, the $A_2 - P_2$ interval narrows, whereas the $A_2 - OS$ interval widens.

Another characteristic is that the $A_2 - OS$ interval remains constant throughout respiration, whereas the

Auscultatory area for opening snap

Mitral area

$A_2 - P_2$ interval normally widens during inspiration and narrows during expiration. During inspiration, three distinct sounds can usually be heard over the pulmonic area; therefore, the sequence must be A_2, P_2, OS. In contrast, during expiration, the $A_2 - P_2$ interval narrows or fuses, forming one sound. This creates an $S_2 - OS$ interval.

Finally, P_2 is not usually heard over the mitral area. Therefore, if you hear a split S_2 over this area, it's likely to be an S_2 and an OS.

Differentiating an OS from S_3

Distinguishing an OS from an S_3 is difficult in some patients, especially in those with mild mitral stenosis when the $A_2 - OS$ interval is wider than usual and the OS is somewhat softer. One characteristic of an OS that helps distinguish it from an S_3 is its timing: The $A_2 - S_3$ interval is usually longer than the $A_2 - OS$ interval. Also, S_3 is a low-frequency sound heard best over the mitral area with the bell of the stethoscope. In contrast, an OS produces a high-frequency sound that's more widely transmitted across the precordium and is heard best with the diaphragm.

Another characteristic of an OS is that its intensity usually isn't affected by having the patient stand, whereas S_2 intensity can be decreased by standing. If the OS is affected, it's intensified. Finally, if the murmur typically heard in patients with mitral stenosis is present, you can confirm that the sound is an OS.

⊚ **AUSCULTATION TIP** S_3 is usually louder during expiration than during inspiration and is often palpable; an OS doesn't vary in intensity with respiration.

Area producing ejection sound

1. Stenotic aortic valve
2. Stenotic pulmonic valve

Systolic ejection sounds

Just as an OS is caused by stenotic mitral valve leaflets, a systolic ejection sound (ES) is caused by the opening of a stenotic aortic or pulmonic valve.

A systolic ES usually occurs early in systole after S_1 and isovolumic contraction. It's commonly associated with ventricular ejection and the maximum opening of a stenotic, yet mobile, aortic or pulmonic valve. If the valve is severely stenotic because of calcification, a systolic ES — like an OS — won't be produced. A systolic ES is considered an abnormal condition whether it originates in the heart's right or left side. It may also be caused by sudden distention of an already dilated aorta or pulmonary artery and by forceful ventricular ejection from pulmonary or systemic hypertension.

Auscultatory area and relationship to ECG

A systolic ES is usually a brief, high-frequency sound that's heard best with the diaphragm of the stethoscope. It may be heard near the heart's base over the aortic or pulmonic area, over Erb's point, or near the apex near the mitral area. A systolic ES occurs just after the QRS complex in the ECG waveform.

Pulmonic ejection sounds

A pulmonic ejection sound (PES), heard best over the pulmonic area, is the only right-sided heart sound that increases in intensity during expiration and diminishes or disappears during inspiration. (♦37____) In a normal heart, inspiration increases right ventricular volume, causing the pulmonic valve to dome toward the pulmonary artery, which decreases the sound's intensity. During expiration, right ventricular volume is decreased, the valve is less domed, and its opening produces a louder snap. In a patient with pulmonary artery dilation or pulmonary hypertension, a PES may not vary in intensity during respiration.

SOUND CHARACTERISTICS
A PES is usually heard best near the heart's base over the pulmonic area. Its intensity is soft but may be equal to or greater than that of S_1; it has a short duration. It has a high pitch heard best with the diaphragm of the stethoscope and a sharp, or clicklike, quality. Its timing is closely related to S_1. A PES occurs early in ventricular systole, just after the opening of a stenotic pulmonic valve (♦38____), and is heard just after the QRS complex.

 AUSCULTATION TIP To differentiate between a PES and an S_1, remember that a PES is heard in the pulmonic area and varies with respiration, whereas a split S_1 is heard in the tricuspid area and doesn't vary with respiration.

Using a PES to differentiate clinical conditions

Because a PES may occur in idiopathic dilation of the pulmonary artery, but is usually not present in supravalvular or muscular subvalvular obstructions, its presence can be used to differentiate between these conditions. Occa-

Auscultatory area for pulmonic ejection sound

Pulmonic area

PCG and ECG showing pulmonic ejection sound

Inspiration   Expiration

Auscultatory area for aortic ejection sound

1. Mitral area
2. Erb's point
3. Aortic area

sionally, a PES may also be heard with atrial and ventricular septal defects.

Aortic ejection sounds

An aortic ejection sound (AES) is heard best near the heart's apex over the mitral area, near the heart's base over the aortic area, or over Erb's point. (♦39____) An AES may be heard in patients with aortic stenosis or aortic insufficiency, but the sound is less clicklike when associated with aortic insufficiency.

Unlike a PES, caused by pulmonic valve stenosis, an AES, caused by aortic valve stenosis, does not vary in intensity with respiration. An AES may occur in patients with aortic root dilation, which is commonly associated with such conditions as systemic hypertension, an ascending aortic aneurysm, or coarctation of the aorta.

SOUND CHARACTERISTICS

An AES is heard best near the heart's apex over the mitral area, near the heart's base over the aortic area, or over Erb's point. Its intensity is soft but may be equal to or greater than that of S_1. An AES has a short duration. It has a high pitch that is heard best with the diaphragm of the stethoscope and a sharp, or clicklike, quality. Its timing is closely related to S_1. (♦40____) An AES occurs early in ventricular systole, just after the opening of a stenot-

PCG and ECG showing aortic ejection sound

ic aortic valve, and is heard just after the QRS complex in the ECG waveform.

Differentiating an AES from other heart sounds

Certain characteristics help to distinguish an AES from other heart sounds. One characteristic is that an AES radiates more than a PES. Another characteristic is that a split S_1 heard over the mitral area is likely to be an M_1 and an AES.

You can differentiate an AES from an S_4 by remembering that S_4 is heard best with the bell of the stethoscope over the mitral area and is frequently accompanied by a palpable, presystolic apical bulge. Also, an S_4 is intensified by maneuvers that increase venous return to the heart, such as brief exercise, squatting, raising the legs from a recumbent position, coughing, or performing Valsalva's maneuver; an AES isn't affected by any of these maneuvers.

Clicks

An MSC occurs when the prolapsed mitral valve's leaflets and chordae tendineae tense. The anterior or posterior leaflet or both leaflets can prolapse. Occasionally, multiple clicks occur that are heard in mid- to late systole; they are heard best over the tricuspid area and toward the mitral area. Like ejection sounds, these mid- to late systolic clicks are crisp, high-frequency sounds. (♦41_____)

Area producing midsystolic click

Prolapsed mitral valve ⎯

PCG and ECG showing midsystolic click

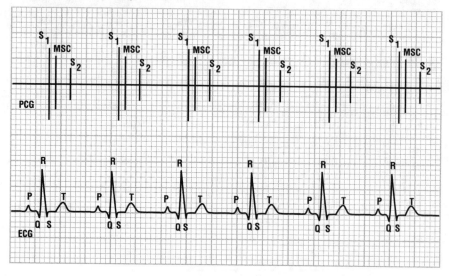

Auscultatory area for midsystolic click

1. Tricuspid area
2. Mitral area

SOUND CHARACTERISTICS

An MSC is usually heard best over the tricuspid area and near the heart's apex over the mitral area. Its intensity is equal to or greater than that of S_1. An MSC has a short duration. It has a high pitch that is heard best with the diaphragm of the stethoscope, and its quality is clicklike. The click's timing varies; it can occur in early, mid-, or late systole. An MSC can be heard during the QT interval in the ECG waveform. (◆42___)

Differentiating an MSC from other heart sounds

The timing of an MSC is affected by various maneuvers, such as having the patient stand or perform Valsalva's maneuver. Such maneuvers result in reduced left ventricular filling and cause the MSC to be heard closer to S_1. The MSC may even merge with S_1 and disappear completely. Increasing left ventricular volume by raising the legs from a recumbent position delays the click. This maneuver may also cause the prolapse not to occur and the MSC to be diminished or inaudible.

Sometimes an MSC is accompanied by a late systolic crescendo murmur or the characteristic holosystolic murmur of mitral regurgitation. An MSC may also be caused by some extracardiac conditions such as pleuropericardial adhesions, atrial septal aneurysms, and cardiac tumors.

◤ POSTTEST

1. What heart sound is produced when the mitral valve leaflets become stenotic or abnormally narrowed?
2. Describe the characteristics of an opening snap (OS).
3. How can you tell the difference between an OS and S_2?
4. How can you tell the difference between an OS and S_3?
5. What is a systolic ejection sound?
6. What causes a pulmonic ejection sound (PES)?
7. Describe the characteristics of a PES.
8. What is the primary difference between a PES and an aortic ejection sound (AES)?
9. Describe the characteristics of an AES.
10. How can you tell the difference between an AES and other heart sounds?
11. What causes a midsystolic click (MSC)?
12. Describe the characteristics of an MSC.
13. How can you tell the difference between an MSC and other heart sounds?

16

Murmur fundamentals

▶❚❙ *PRETEST*
1. How does turbulent blood flow produce murmurs?
2. What are the seven characteristics used to describe murmurs?
3. What is the six-point graded scale?
4. What is a murmur's configuration?

Turbulent blood flow

Whereas heart sounds are produced by brief vibrations that correspond to the beginning and end of systole, murmurs are produced by a prolonged series of vibrations that occurs during systole, diastole, or both. These vibrations result from turbulent blood flow.

Several clinically significant conditions — such as blood flowing at a high velocity through a partially obstructed opening, blood flowing from a smaller chamber to a larger one, or any combination of these — can cause turbulent blood flow.

Characteristics

Murmurs, like other heart sounds, are described by their audible characteristics heard during auscultation. The terms used to describe a specific characteristic are determined primarily by the volume and speed of the jet of blood as it moves through the heart.

The seven characteristics used to describe murmurs are location, intensity, duration, pitch, quality, timing, and configuration.

AUSCULTATION TIP Initially, learn to identify the location and timing of murmurs. As your auscultation techniques improve, try to identify the intensity, duration, pitch, quality, and configuration.

A murmur's *location* is the anatomic area on the chest wall where the murmur is heard best and is usually also the murmur's point of maximum intensity. This area usually correlates with the underlying location of the valve that is responsible for producing the murmur. For example, an aortic stenosis murmur is usually heard best near the heart's base over the aortic area, whereas a mitral regurgitation murmur is usually heard best near the heart's apex over the mitral area.

The murmur's sounds may also be transmitted to the chamber or vessel where the turbulent blood flow occurs. This phenomenon, known as *radiation,* occurs because the direction of blood flow determines sound transmission. Murmurs radiate in either a forward or a backward direction.

The second characteristic, *intensity,* refers to the murmur's loudness. Intensity is influenced by many factors, including body weight. For example, because transmission of heart sounds to the chest wall is affected by chest wall thickness and by certain diseases, heart sounds and murmurs are usually louder in thin individuals and fainter in obese individuals. They are also fainter in patients with emphysema.

Hyperdynamic states, decreased blood viscosity, increased pressure gradients across valves, larger jets of blood, and faster heart rates may also increase a murmur's intensity. Murmurs are less intense in hypodynamic states and in patients with an elevated hematocrit.

Document a murmur's intensity using a uniform method. Most health care professionals use a six-point graded scale, with 1 being the faintest intensity and 6 being the loudest. A grade 1 murmur is faint, may be heard intermittently, and is barely heard through the stethoscope. A grade 2 murmur is also faint but is usually heard as soon as the stethoscope is placed on the chest wall. A grade 3 murmur is easily heard and is described as moderately loud. A grade 4 murmur is loud and is usually associated with a palpable vibration known as a *thrill.* It also may radiate in the direction of blood flow. A grade 5 murmur is loud enough to be heard with only an edge of the stethoscope touching the chest wall; it's almost always accompanied by a thrill and radiation. A grade 6 murmur is

Crescendo murmur

Decrescendo murmur

Crescendo-decrescendo murmur

Plateau-shaped murmur

so loud that it can be heard with the stethoscope close to, but not touching, the chest wall; it's always accompanied by a thrill, and it radiates to distant structures.

When you document a murmur's grade, write it as a fraction — for example, ⅜. This means you consider it to be a grade 3 and have used the six-point scale for assessment. That way, all health care professionals will understand which scale was used, even if they don't use the same one.

Duration, the length of time the murmur is heard during systole or diastole, may be described as long or short.

A murmur's *pitch,* or frequency, varies from high to low. It's usually higher in conditions accompanied by increased blood flow velocity or increased pressure gradients and lower in conditions associated with lower blood flow velocity. Blood flow through narrowed valves or vessels also usually increases pitch.

A murmur's *quality* is determined by the combination of frequencies that produces the sound. It's typically described as harsh, rough, musical, scratchy, squeaky, rumbling, or blowing.

A murmur's *timing* refers to when the murmur occurs in the cardiac cycle. This means that the onset, duration, and end of the murmur are described in relation to systole and diastole. The beginning of systole, or S_1, can be identified easily by palpating the carotid pulse or by looking for the QRS complex on the ECG monitor's oscilloscope.

All systolic murmurs occur between S_1 and S_2 during ventricular systole; this interval is between the QRS complex and the T wave in the ECG waveform. All diastolic murmurs occur between S_2 and S_1 during ventricular diastole; this interval is between the T wave and the QRS complex in the ECG waveform.

Murmurs are further classified according to their timing within the phases of the cardiac cycle. For example, a murmur can be described as holosystolic, meaning it's present throughout systole, or as early, mid-, or late systolic or diastolic.

The last characteristic, *configuration,* refers to the shape of a murmur's sound as recorded on a phonocardiogram. The configuration is usually defined by changes in the murmur's intensity during systole or diastole and is determined by blood flow pressure gradients. For example, a crescendo murmur is one that gradually increases in intensity as the pressure gradient increases. A decrescendo murmur is one that gradually decreases in intensity as the pressure gradient decreases. A crescendo-decrescendo murmur first increases in intensity as the pressure gradient increases, then decreases in intensity as the pressure gradient decreases; it's also known as a diamond-shaped murmur. Finally, a plateau-shaped murmur is one that is equal in intensity throughout the murmur.

Murmurs must be described carefully and accurately using these seven characteristics. Making such information immediately available to all that care for a specific patient will allow any changes in a murmur's characteristics to be recognized easily. In that way, the possible source of those changes can be assessed more easily.

POSTTEST

1. What causes turbulent blood flow?
2. What determines a murmur's sound characteristics?
3. List the seven characteristics used to describe murmurs.
4. What is a murmur's location?
5. What does the term radiation mean?
6. What is a murmur's intensity?
7. Describe the six-point graded scale.
8. What is a murmur's duration?
9. What is a murmur's pitch?
10. What is a murmur's quality?
11. What is a murmur's timing?
12. What is a murmur's configuration?
13. What are the four configurations used to describe a murmur?

17

Systolic murmurs

▶️ PRETEST

1. How is the sound of a systolic murmur produced?
2. What are ventricular outflow obstruction murmurs?
3. List the murmurs associated with right ventricular outflow obstruction.
4. List the murmurs associated with left ventricular outflow obstruction.
5. How is the sound of a systolic regurgitation murmur produced?
6. List the systolic regurgitation murmurs.

Anatomy and physiology

Area producing systolic ejection murmur

1. Aortic valve
2. Pulmonic valve
3. Right ventricle
4. Left ventricle

Normally, as ventricular pressures rise at the beginning of systole, the mitral and tricuspid valves close. Then, for a brief time, while the aortic and pulmonic valves are still closed during isovolumic contraction, ventricular pressures rise sharply. When the pressure in both ventricles is high enough, the aortic and pulmonic valves open, and blood is ejected from the ventricles into the aorta and the pulmonary artery. Normally, functioning valves facilitate this unidirectional blood flow.

However, aortic or pulmonic outlet abnormalities may generate forward systolic ejection murmurs. When the mitral or tricuspid valve is involved, backward, or regurgitant, murmurs may be heard during systole. All systolic murmurs occur during ventricular systole between S_1 and S_2.

Systolic ejection murmurs

During ventricular systole, the rapid ejection of blood from the ventricles causes turbulent blood flow, which produces an innocent systolic ejection murmur (SEM). (♦43____) This murmur, which is present in all people and is considered to be normal, is usually inaudible. However, in thin-chested individuals, children, and patients with hyperdynamic states, such as anemia, thyrotoxicosis, fever, pregnancy, or arteriovenous shunts, an SEM can often be auscultated.

An SEM, classified as benign or functional, is called an *innocent* or *flow murmur* because it isn't caused by an obstruction. However, unusual turbulence related to dilatation of the aorta or pulmonary artery may also produce an innocent SEM. Medical researchers believe such SEMs are caused by sclerotic changes in the aortic valve cusps. Approximately 50% of all persons over age 50 have this type of murmur, which is heard more commonly in women and in patients with hypertension.

SOUND CHARACTERISTICS
An SEM is usually heard best along the left sternal border and sometimes over the aortic and mitral areas. Its intensity is usually soft (less than a grade ⅚), and the duration of the intensity is short.

 AUSCULTATION TIP To determine if a murmur intensifies, listen at the murmur's border.

An SEM has a medium pitch heard best with the diaphragm of the stethoscope. The quality of an SEM is variable. Its timing is early systolic; it ends well before a normal S_2 split. It's heard after the QRS complex in the electrocardiogram (ECG) waveform. (See *PCG and ECG showing systolic ejection murmur,* page 140.) An SEM has a crescendo-decrescendo configuration. (♦44____)

Auscultatory area for systolic ejection murmur

1. Left sternal border
2. Aortic area
3. Mitral area

ENHANCEMENT TECHNIQUES
An SEM's intensity can be increased by maneuvers that increase blood volume or ejection velocity, such as having the patient raise his legs from a recumbent position, exercise briefly, or cough a few times.

PCG and ECG showing systolic ejection murmur

Ventricular outflow obstruction murmurs

Right or left ventricular outflow obstructions may be supravalvular, valvular, or subvalvular. Regardless of location, the outflow obstruction causes turbulent blood flow, which produces a midsystolic ejection murmur. The murmur begins early in systole — after S_1 and the opening of the diseased pulmonic or aortic valve. It ends before the S_2 closure component of the diseased pulmonic or aortic valve. This murmur typically has a crescendo-decrescendo configuration that peaks in intensity in early, mid-, or late systole, depending on the severity of the obstruction.

Right ventricular outflow obstruction murmurs

Supravalvular pulmonic stenosis murmurs

Supravalvular pulmonic stenosis, or pulmonary artery branch stenosis, is a type of right ventricular outflow obstruction that occurs above the pulmonic valve. This obstruction produces a murmur with a crescendo-decrescendo configuration that is occasionally continuous. (♦45____) The murmur is rarely accompanied by a pulmonic ejection sound (PES) but is associated with a P_2 of normal intensity.

Area producing supravalvular pulmonic stenosis murmur

Supravalvular pulmonic area —

PCG and ECG showing supravalvular pulmonic stenosis murmur

SOUND CHARACTERISTICS

The supravalvular pulmonic stenosis murmur is usually heard over much of the thorax. Its intensity and duration are variable. It has a medium pitch heard best with the diaphragm of the stethoscope and a harsh quality. Its timing is systolic: It begins after S_1 and ends before a normal S_2 split. In the ECG waveform, the murmur begins just after the QRS complex begins and ends just before the T wave ends. It has a crescendo-decrescendo configuration that is occasionally continuous. (♦46____)

Auscultatory area for supravalvular pulmonic stenosis murmur

Pulmonic valvular stenosis murmurs

The pulmonic valvular stenosis murmur results from congenital pulmonic valvular stenosis and is often associated with other congenital defects. In mild pulmonic valvular stenosis, S_1 is normal. The murmur begins after S_1 with a right-sided PES as the pulmonic valve abruptly stops opening. Remember, the PES is the only right-sided heart sound that increases in intensity during expiration and becomes less audible during inspiration. The murmur intensifies after the PES and peaks in midsystole; then it begins to fade. It ends before S_2. The intensity of P_2 is normal. (♦47____)

In severe pulmonic valvular stenosis, the pressure gradient across the pulmonic valve increases. An increased pressure gradient causes the PES to be heard earlier; it may even fuse with S_1. Right ventricular ejection time is also pro-

Area producing pulmonic valvular stenosis murmur

Pulmonic valvular area

PCG and ECG showing pulmonic valvular stenosis murmur

longed. Consequently, the murmur has a longer crescendo and the intensity peaks later in systole. It continues throughout A_1 but ends before P_2. Prolonged right ventricular ejection time also causes a delayed P_2, creating a wide S_2 split.

Usually, as the stenosis becomes more severe, the murmur's duration lengthens and its configuration becomes more asymmetrical. Consequently, P_2 is delayed even more and its intensity is decreased.

SOUND CHARACTERISTICS

The pulmonic valvular stenosis murmur is heard best near the heart's base over the pulmonic area. It often radiates toward the left neck or the left shoulder. The murmur's intensity is usually soft, but it will become louder with a palpable thrill toward the left neck and shoulder as the stenosis becomes more severe. Its duration is short, but this too will increase as the stenosis worsens. It has a medium pitch heard best with the diaphragm of the stethoscope and a harsh quality. Its timing is midsystolic: It ends before a normal S_2 split. It's accompanied by a PES that diminishes or disappears with inspiration. In the ECG waveform, it begins after the QRS complex and ends before the end of the T wave. The murmur has a crescendo-decrescendo configuration. A mild pulmonic valvular stenosis murmur is shaped like a diamond; a severe pulmonic valvular stenosis murmur is shaped like a kite. (♦48____)

Auscultatory area for pulmonic valvular stenosis murmur

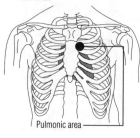

Pulmonic area

PCG and ECG showing subvalvular pulmonic stenosis murmur

Subvalvular pulmonic stenosis murmurs

When a right ventricular outflow obstruction is beneath the pulmonic valve, or subvalvular, the midsystolic ejection murmur sounds the same as a pulmonic valvular stenosis murmur. However, it isn't initiated by a PES. (♦49____) If the subvalvular obstruction is associated with a ventricular septal defect, the murmur will be more complex in character.

SOUND CHARACTERISTICS

The subvalvular pulmonic stenosis murmur is usually heard best over the pulmonic area and over Erb's point; it often radiates toward the left side of the neck, the left shoulder, or both. Its intensity is usually soft but becomes louder as the stenosis worsens. The duration, which is short, also increases as the stenosis worsens. The murmur has a medium pitch heard best with the diaphragm of the stethoscope; its quality is harsh. Its timing is midsystolic: It starts after S_1 and ends before a normal S_2 split. On an ECG, the murmur begins after the QRS complex and ends before the end of the T wave. (♦50____) This murmur isn't initiated by a PES. It has a crescendo-decrescendo configuration.

Area producing subvalvular pulmonic stenosis murmur

Subvalvular pulmonic area

Auscultatory area for subvalvular pulmonic stenosis murmur

1. Pulmonic area
2. Erb's point

PCG and ECG showing supravalvular aortic stenosis murmur

Area producing supraval-vular aortic stenosis murmur

Supravalvular aortic area

Auscultatory area for supraval-vular aortic stenosis murmur

1. Suprasternal notch
2. First intercostal space
3. Aortic area

Left ventricular outflow obstruction murmurs
Supravalvular aortic stenosis murmurs

When a left ventricular outflow obstruction is above the aortic valve, or supravalvular, it produces a murmur with a crescendo-decrescendo configuration. (♦51____) Supravalvular aortic stenosis is usually congenital. Its characteristics are similar to those of aortic valvular stenosis, except that it has no aortic ejection sound (AES), is louder, and is heard best over the suprasternal area, aortic area, or right first intercostal space.

SOUND CHARACTERISTICS

The supravalvular aortic stenosis murmur is usually heard best near the heart's base over the right first intercostal space, over the aortic area, and over the suprasternal notch. It may radiate toward the right side of the neck, the right shoulder, or both. Its intensity, typically a grade ⅜ to ⅘, decreases in patients with left ventricular failure. Its duration increases as the stenosis worsens. It has a medium pitch that can be heard equally well with the diaphragm or bell of the stethoscope. The murmur has a rough quality. Its timing is midsystolic: It ends before a normal S_2 split. It isn't associated with an AES. In the ECG waveform, it begins after the QRS complex and ends before the end of the T wave. The murmur has a crescendo-decrescendo configuration. (♦52____)

Aortic valvular stenosis murmurs

Aortic valvular stenosis may be congenital or may be acquired from degenerative or rheumatic heart disease. If it's acquired from rheumatic heart disease, the mitral valve is commonly affected as well. Aortic stenosis produces an SEM that begins after S_1 and ends before S_2. (♦53____) After S_1, left ventricular pressure rises. The stenotic aortic valve halts its opening motion and produces a loud AES heard best near the heart's apex over the mitral area. The AES is followed by the murmur, which gradually intensifies until mid- to late systole and then fades, ending before a faint A_2.

When an aortic valvular stenosis murmur is discovered late in adulthood, it can be heard best over the mitral area. As the valve becomes more calcified with age, and consequently less mobile, both the AES and A_2 become soft or even inaudible. The murmur can vary in intensity from a soft grade ⅖ to a rough grade ⁴⁄₆ sound, but most aortic valvular stenosis murmurs are a grade ⅗ to ⁴⁄₆.

SOUND CHARACTERISTICS

The aortic valvular stenosis murmur is usually heard best near the heart's base over the aortic area, over Erb's point, near the heart's apex over the mitral area, or over the suprasternal notch. The murmur may radiate toward the right side of the neck, the right shoulder, or both. A thrill may be palpable over the aortic area and neck. The murmur's intensity, typically a grade ⅗ to ⁴⁄₆, decreases in patients with left ventricular failure. Its duration increases as stenosis worsens.

The aortic valvular stenosis murmur has a medium pitch heard equally well with the diaphragm or bell of the stethoscope. The murmur's quality is rough and may become harsher and louder as stenosis worsens. Its timing is midsystolic. An AES, when present, is heard shortly after S_1; the AES is followed by the murmur, which ends before a normal S_1 split. If an S_4 is heard before age 40, stenosis is usually severe. In the ECG waveform, the murmur begins after the QRS complex and ends before the end of the T wave. It has a crescendo-decrescendo configuration. (♦54____)

Area producing aortic valvular stenosis murmur

Aortic valvular area ┘

Auscultatory area for aortic valvular stenosis murmur

1. Suprasternal notch
2. Aortic area
3. Erb's point
4. Mitral area

PCG and ECG showing aortic valvular stenosis murmur

VARIATIONS

Certain characteristics of the aortic valvular stenosis murmur vary according to the degree of stenosis. For example, as stenosis worsens, left ventricular ejection time is prolonged, and the murmur peaks later in systole. A delayed A_2 and a shortened $A_2 - P_2$ interval are also heard.

Also, the more severe the stenosis, the closer A_2 moves to P_2. With extremely severe stenosis, A_2 becomes soft and actually follows P_2, producing a paradoxical S_2 split.

Subvalvular aortic stenosis murmurs

When a left ventricular outflow obstruction is below the aortic valve, or subvalvular, it produces a murmur with a crescendo-decrescendo configuration. ($\blacklozenge$ 55____) A subvalvular aortic outflow obstruction may be caused by a congenital fibrous ring, or it may be acquired from hypertrophic cardiomyopathy (formerly known as idiopathic hypertrophic subaortic stenosis). This is a dynamic obstruction produced by asymmetrical hypertrophy of the septum and an abnormal anterior motion of the mitral valve leaflets during systole.

Area producing subvalvular aortic stenosis murmur

Subvalvular aortic area

SOUND CHARACTERISTICS

The subvalvular aortic stenosis murmur is usually heard best near the heart's apex over the mitral and tricuspid areas. It doesn't usually radiate toward the base, right side of the neck, or right shoulder. Its intensity, typically a grade

PCG and ECG showing subvalvular aortic stenosis murmur

⅜ to ⅘, will increase as stenosis worsens; its duration is variable. The murmur has a medium pitch that is heard equally well with the bell or diaphragm of the stethoscope. Its quality can be harsh or rough. This murmur's timing is midsystolic: It peaks in midsystole and ends before a normal S_2 split, a delayed A_2, or a paradoxical S_2 split. In the ECG waveform, it begins after the QRS complex and ends before the end of the T wave. The murmur has a crescendo-decrescendo configuration. (♦56___)

Differentiating subvalvular and aortic valvular stenosis murmurs

A subvalvular hypertrophic cardiomyopathic murmur becomes louder during Valsalva's maneuver, whereas an aortic valvular stenosis murmur does not. Performing Valsalva's maneuver or having the patient stand up suddenly decreases venous return and left ventricular filling; this makes the left ventricle smaller, the obstruction more severe, and the subvalvular hypertrophic cardiomyopathic murmur louder. Having the patient squat increases peripheral vascular resistance and left ventricular filling; this maneuver decreases the pressure gradient across the aortic valve and decreases or obliterates the subvalvular hypertrophic cardiomyopathic murmur.

Auscultatory area for subvalvular aortic stenosis murmur

1. Tricuspid area
2. Mitral area

Systolic regurgitation murmurs

An abnormality of either the tricuspid or mitral valve may result in backward turbulent blood flow during systole. This means that blood moves in a direction opposite that of the normal unidirectional flow pattern. Blood regurgitates through a defective, incompetent tricuspid or mitral valve into the left or right atrium, resulting in what is commonly called tricuspid or mitral valve insufficiency. An incompetent valve may be caused by a primary valvular disorder or may develop secondary to dysfunction of the valve's supporting structures.

The regurgitant murmurs heard in patients with these disorders may be early or late systolic, or holosystolic. The early systolic murmurs have a crescendo-decrescendo configuration, the late systolic murmurs have either a crescendo or crescendo-decrescendo configuration, and the holosystolic murmurs have a plateau shape.

Tricuspid regurgitation murmurs

The tricuspid regurgitation murmur, also called tricuspid insufficiency, most often results from right ventricular dilation, which usually results from mitral valve disease or left ventricular failure but may also be caused by pulmonary disease. It occasionally results from a congenital valve malformation and may also be acquired as a result of infective endocarditis, a right ventricular infarction, or trauma to the valve or its supporting structures.

This murmur can also be heard occasionally in a patient with a transvenous pacemaker because the pacemaker lead interferes with tricuspid valve closure, creating a tricuspid regurgitation-type murmur. The T_1 (tricuspid valve closure) intensity is either increased, normal, or decreased. ($\blacklozenge$ 57_____)

SOUND CHARACTERISTICS
The tricuspid regurgitation murmur is usually heard best over the tricuspid area; in some patients, it's heard only during inspiration. The murmur may radiate to the right of the sternum. Its usually soft intensity may increase during deep inspiration. The murmur's duration is long. It has a high pitch heard best with the diaphragm of the stethoscope and a scratchy or blowing quality. The murmur's timing is systolic: It lasts from S_1 to P_2. In the ECG waveform, the mur-

Area producing tricuspid regurgitation murmur

Regurgitant tricuspid valve

PCG and ECG showing tricuspid regurgitation murmur

mur begins just after the QRS complex and ends after the T wave. It is holosystolic and plateau-shaped. (♦58____)

ENHANCEMENT TECHNIQUES

Regardless of the tricuspid regurgitation murmur's etiology, the murmur increases in intensity during inspiration because venous return and right ventricular filling are increased, creating higher pressure gradients during systole. To enhance the murmur, have the patient breathe through his mouth slowly, quietly, and deeply while sitting or standing. Caution the patient not to hold his breath because this negates the maneuver's effect. Another technique is to apply pressure inward and upward below the right costal margin. The murmur is louder during inspiration. In some patients, this is the only time the murmur is audible.

If the tricuspid regurgitation murmur is secondary to right ventricular failure, right ventricular filling may be limited with inspiration; consequently, the murmur may not be intensified during deep breathing.

This murmur is rarely accompanied by a systolic thrill, and neither its timing in systole nor its intensity correlates with the severity of the regurgitation.

Auscultatory area for tricuspid regurgitation murmur

Tricuspid area

Area producing mitral regurgitation murmur

Regurgitant mitral valve

Auscultatory area for mitral regurgitation murmur

Mitral area

Mitral regurgitation murmurs

The mitral regurgitation murmur, also called mitral insufficiency, may be caused by a congenital or acquired abnormality of the mitral valve leaflets, the valve's supporting structures, or the left ventricle. An incompetent mitral valve causes backward blood flow through the incompetent mitral valve during systole. The increased resistance at the aortic valve facilitates regurgitation of blood through the incompetent mitral valve into the left atrium, producing the mitral regurgitation murmur. (♦59____)

This murmur may appear in early, mid-, or late systole, or it may be holosystolic. Its quality, duration, and radiation depend on the extent, duration, and location of the disease process. Usually, late systolic murmurs are associated with mild to moderate regurgitation.

Holosystolic mitral regurgitation murmurs

The holosystolic mitral regurgitation murmur can be caused by the effects of rheumatic heart disease on the mitral valve, by mitral valve prolapse, by left ventricular dilation, or by papillary muscle dysfunction. The murmur can usually be heard regardless of the patient's position, but grade ⅙ to ⅖ murmurs may be heard better with the patient in the partial left lateral recumbent position or after exercise.

A loud S_3 usually accompanies moderate to severe mitral regurgitation; this sound is related not to ventricular failure but to the increased left ventricular volume in early diastole.

SOUND CHARACTERISTICS

The holosystolic mitral regurgitation murmur is usually heard best near the heart's apex over the mitral area. The sound may radiate to the axilla or posteriorly over the lung bases. Its intensity is variable and usually not affected by respiration; however, it may be somewhat diminished during inspiration. The murmur has a long duration. It has a medium to high pitch heard best with the diaphragm of the stethoscope. The murmur may be accompanied by a systolic apical thrill. Its quality is blowing, and its timing is systolic — from S_1 to S_2. In the ECG waveform, it's heard from just after the QRS complex to the end of the T wave. The murmur is holosystolic and plateau-shaped. (♦60____)

PCG and ECG showing mitral regurgitation murmur

Acute mitral regurgitation murmurs

Acute mitral regurgitation is less common than chronic mitral regurgitation. Its murmur results from rupture of the chordae tendineae, papillary muscle, or both. Occasionally, this murmur occurs with a myocardial infarction, but it may also result from severe damage to the mitral valve from trauma or infection.

ALERT Rupture of the chordae tendineae may lead to acute pulmonary edema. Notify the doctor immediately, and monitor the patient for signs and symptoms of acute pulmonary edema (acute shortage of breath, rapid respiration, audible wheezes and crackles, productive cough that produces a frothy, blood-tinged sputum; tachycardia, hypotension, and cyanotic, cold, clammy skin).

The acute mitral regurgitation murmur begins with mitral valve closure and is holosystolic. (♦61____) However, its intensity decreases as ventricular and atrial pressures equilibrate during late systole. S_3 and S_4 are usually heard in acute mitral regurgitation.

SOUND CHARACTERISTICS

The acute mitral regurgitation murmur is usually heard best near the heart's apex over the mitral area. Its intensity is usually loud (grade ⁴⁄₆ to ⁶⁄₆ if the murmur results from rupture of the chordae tendineae). It's accompanied

Auscultatory area for acute mitral regurgitation murmur

Mitral area

PCG and ECG showing acute mitral regurgitation murmur

by a systolic thrill. The murmur's duration is long. It has a high pitch heard best with the diaphragm of the stethoscope and a quality that can be musical. Its timing is systolic: It begins with M_1 and ends with or before A_2. In the ECG waveform, the murmur begins just after the QRS complex and ends just after the T wave. It's holosystolic and wedge-shaped (the wedge shape has a steeper decrescendo configuration). (◆62____)

Mitral valve prolapse murmurs

Mitral valve prolapse is one of the most common valvular abnormalities found in adults. The murmur associated with a prolapsed mitral valve usually appears in late systole and is either isolated or accompanied by a nonejection midsystolic click or clicks caused by the mitral valve prolapsing and ballooning up into the left atrium. This is sometimes referred to as the click-murmur syndrome. (◆63____)

Area producing mitral valve prolapse murmur

Prolapsed mitral valve

SOUND CHARACTERISTICS

The mitral valve prolapse murmur is usually heard best near the heart's apex over the mitral area. Its intensity is usually soft (grade ⅖ to ⅗), and its duration is short. It has a high pitch heard best with the diaphragm of the stethoscope. The murmur has a musical quality; when loud, it's sometimes described as a whoop or honk. Its timing is usually late systolic but can sometimes be holosys-

PCG and ECG showing mitral valve prolapse murmur

tolic. In the ECG waveform, the murmur coincides with the T wave and ends just after the T wave. It has a crescendo or crescendo-decrescendo configuration. ($\blacklozenge$64_____)

ENHANCEMENT TECHNIQUES

Having the patient stand decreases left ventricular volume, which causes the mitral valve prolapse murmur to be heard earlier in systole, to be louder, and to last longer. Having the patient squat increases left ventricular volume, which causes the murmur to be heard later in systole.

The direction in which the mitral valve prolapse murmur is transmitted across the chest wall depends on the disease process. For example, if the mitral valve's posterior leaflet is involved, blood flow might be directed more anteriorly and medially. Consequently, the murmur would be transmitted toward the heart's base and heard best over the aortic area and along the left sternal edge. If the anterior leaflet is incompetent, blood flow is directed posteriorly against the posterior left atrial wall, and the murmur is transmitted toward the left axilla and back.

Auscultatory area for mitral valve prolapse murmur

Mitral area

PCG and ECG showing a ventricular septal defect murmur

Area producing ventricular septal defect murmur

Ventricular septal defect murmur

A ventricular septal defect (VSD) is an opening, usually in the membranous portion of the ventricular septum, that allows direct communication between the ventricles. Typically, blood shunts from left to right because of higher pressures in the left ventricle.

SOUND CHARACTERISTICS

The VSD murmur is heard over the lower sternal border and, if loud, can be heard over the entire precordium. A thrill may be palpable along the lower left sternal border. The murmur is holosystolic. S_2 is widely split as the aortic valve closes early. If the VSD is very large, pulmonary hypertension eventually develops, the S_2 narrows, and the P_2 becomes louder than the A_2. The intensity and pitch vary with the size of the VSD. If pulmonary hypertension becomes severe, shunting may stop and the P_2 and A_2 may merge.

◪ *POSTTEST*

1. Describe the sound production of systolic murmurs.
2. How is the sound of an innocent systolic ejection murmur (SEM) produced?
3. Describe the characteristics of an SEM.
4. How can an SEM be enhanced?
5. What is a ventricular outflow obstruction murmur?
6. Describe the characteristics of a supravalvular pulmonic stenosis murmur.
7. Compare mild pulmonic valvular stenosis with severe pulmonic valvular stenosis.
8. Describe the characteristics of a pulmonic valvular stenosis murmur.
9. Describe the characteristics of a subvalvular pulmonic stenosis murmur.
10. Describe the characteristics of a supravalvular aortic stenosis murmur.
11. Describe the characteristics of an aortic valvular stenosis murmur.
12. What causes subvalvular aortic stenosis?
13. Describe the characteristics of a subvalvular aortic stenosis murmur.
14. How are systolic regurgitation murmurs produced?
15. Describe the characteristics of a tricuspid regurgitation murmur.
16. How can the tricuspid regurgitation murmur be enhanced?
17. How is the sound of a mitral regurgitation murmur produced?
18. Describe the characteristics of a holosystolic mitral regurgitation murmur.
19. Describe the characteristics of an acute mitral regurgitation murmur.
20. Describe the characteristics of a mitral valve prolapse murmur.
21. What maneuvers enhance the mitral valve prolapse murmur?

18

Diastolic murmurs

▶❙❙ *PRETEST*

1. How is the sound of a diastolic murmur produced?
2. List the aortic regurgitation murmurs.
3. List the pulmonic regurgitation murmurs.
4. What are the characteristics of a mitral stenosis murmur?
5. What are the characteristics of a tricuspid stenosis murmur?

At the end of ventricular systole and the beginning of diastole, the aortic and pulmonic valves close. During this time, the $A_2 - P_2$ interval can usually be auscultated. After a brief period of isovolumic relaxation, the mitral and tricuspid valves open and blood flows from the atria into the ventricles. During this early filling period, an S_3 can sometimes be heard in healthy individuals under age 40. Late in diastole, the atria contract, increasing blood flow into the ventricles. Occasionally, an S_4 can be heard during this late filling period. Except for these brief heart sounds, diastole is normally silent. When diastolic murmurs occur, they are heard between S_2 and S_1 or between the end of the T wave and the beginning of the QRS complex in the electrocardiogram (ECG) waveform.

The regurgitation of blood through the aortic and pulmonic valves may cause diastolic murmurs. Since both valves close at the beginning of diastole, murmurs produced by dysfunctional aortic and pulmonic valves begin early in diastole, immediately after the affected valve closes.

Mitral and tricuspid valve stenosis and conditions that produce turbulent blood flow across normal mitral or tricuspid valves also cause diastolic murmurs. Because these valves open after a period of isovolumic relaxation, these murmurs are heard during middiastole.

PCG and ECG showing early diastolic aortic regurgitation murmur

Aortic regurgitation murmurs

Early diastolic aortic regurgitation murmurs

The early diastolic aortic regurgitation murmur, also called aortic insufficiency, can result from rheumatic heart disease, Marfan's syndrome, osteogenesis imperfecta, or a dissecting aortic aneurysm. Leakage around a prosthetic aortic valve can also produce this murmur.

Because aortic pressure normally exceeds left ventricular pressure at the beginning of diastole, it forces a retrograde, or backward, flow of blood across an incompetent aortic valve. The turbulent blood flow produces the murmur. In this murmur, A_2 may sound normal, or it may be accentuated if the patient has severe systemic hypertension. (♦65____) This murmur is commonly associated with a systolic ejection murmur produced by increased left ventricular stroke volume.

SOUND CHARACTERISTICS

The early diastolic aortic regurgitation murmur is usually heard best near the heart's base over the aortic and pulmonic areas, over Erb's point, and near the heart's apex over the mitral area. Because of its usually soft intensity,

Area producing early diastolic aortic regurgitation murmur

Regurgitant aortic valve

Auscultatory area for early diastolic aortic regurgitation murmur

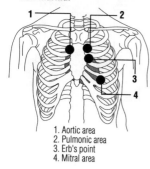

1. Aortic area
2. Pulmonic area
3. Erb's point
4. Mitral area

Area producing middiastolic aortic regurgitation (Austin Flint) murmur

1. Regurgitant aortic valve
2. Anterior mitral leaflet

Auscultatory area for middiastolic aortic regurgitation (Austin Flint) murmur

Mitral area

it's heard best in a quiet environment. The murmur can last throughout most of diastole. It has a high pitch heard best with the diaphragm of the stethoscope and a blowing or musical quality. Its timing is diastolic, beginning with A_2. In the ECG waveform, the murmur begins after the T wave and ends just before the QRS complex. It has a decrescendo configuration. (♦66____)

If aortic regurgitation is associated with aortic root dilation or with a dissecting aneurysm of the ascending aorta, the diastolic murmur may be louder along the right sternal border between the second and fourth intercostal spaces than along the left sternal border between the second and fourth intercostal spaces, respectively. If the patient is elderly or has chronic obstructive pulmonary disease, the murmur may be heard best near the heart's apex over the mitral area. If the murmur is loud, it may be heard over most of the precordium.

ENHANCEMENT TECHNIQUES
This murmur can be enhanced by having the patient sit down, lean forward, and hold his breath after expiration or by maneuvers that increase aortic diastolic pressure, such as having the patient squat.

Middiastolic aortic regurgitation (Austin Flint) murmurs
Severe aortic regurgitation may be associated with a middiastolic and presystolic rumbling murmur. This murmur is caused by the aortic regurgitant jet moving the anterior mitral leaflet toward a closing position, resulting in a relative mitral stenosis. The murmur generated by the turbulent blood flow across the mitral valve is called an Austin Flint murmur. (♦67____)

SOUND CHARACTERISTICS
The Austin Flint murmur is usually heard best near the heart's apex over the mitral area. Its intensity is usually soft. It has a low pitch heard best with the bell of the stethoscope. The murmur has a rumbling quality. Its timing is confined to middiastole or presystole. It's heard just before the QRS complex in the ECG waveform. The murmur has a presystolic crescendo configuration; its middiastolic component has a crescendo-decrescendo configuration. (♦68____)

PCG and ECG showing middiastolic aortic regurgitation (Austin Flint) murmur

Pulmonic regurgitation murmurs

Graham Steell murmurs

Because pulmonary artery pressure is normally quite low during diastole, regurgitation from a normal pulmonic valve rarely occurs without pulmonary hypertension. Pulmonary hypertension produces pulmonary artery dilation and a relative pulmonic insufficiency because of dilation of the pulmonic valve ring. (♦69____) The pulmonic regurgitation murmur resulting from pulmonary hypertension is called a Graham Steell murmur.

SOUND CHARACTERISTICS

The Graham Steell murmur secondary to pulmonary hypertension is usually heard best along the left sternal border over the third and fourth intercostal spaces. It isn't transmitted to the right sternum. Its intensity is usually loud, and its duration is variable. The murmur has a high pitch heard best with the diaphragm of the stethoscope, and it has a blowing quality. Its timing is early diastolic, beginning with a loud P_2. Sometimes an ejection sound can be heard. The murmur is heard after the end of the T wave in the ECG waveform. It has a decrescendo configuration. (♦70____)

Area producing Graham Steell murmur

1. Dilated pulmonary artery
2. Regurgitant pulmonic valve

Auscultatory area for Graham Steell murmur

1. Third intercostal space
2. Fourth intercostal space

PCG and ECG showing Graham Steell murmur

Normal pressure pulmonic valve murmurs

ENHANCEMENT TECHNIQUES
The Graham Steell murmur is intensified during inspiration.

Normal pressure pulmonic valve murmurs

When a murmur results from idiopathic pulmonary artery dilation or congenital pulmonary valve insufficiency, pulmonary artery diastolic pressure isn't elevated. Regurgitation is delayed until right ventricular pressure has fallen below pulmonary artery diastolic pressure during isovolumic relaxation. (♦71____)

SOUND CHARACTERISTICS
The normal pressure pulmonic valve murmur is usually heard best along the left sternal border over the third and fourth intercostal spaces. It isn't transmitted to the right sternum. Its intensity is soft and its duration is brief. The murmur has a low pitch heard best with the bell of the stethoscope. It has a rumbling quality and its timing is early to middiastolic. It begins shortly after P_2 is heard. In the ECG waveform, it begins after the T wave and ends before the P wave. The murmur has a crescendo-decrescendo configuration. (♦72____)

Area producing normal pressure pulmonic valve murmur

1. Dilated pulmonary artery
2. Regurgitant pulmonic valve

PCG and ECG showing normal pressure pulmonic valve murmur

ENHANCEMENT TECHNIQUES

The normal pressure pulmonic valve murmur is intensified during inspiration.

Other diastolic murmurs

Mitral stenosis murmurs

Mitral stenosis results from a congenital defect or chronic rheumatic valvulitis. Typically, valvulitis results in scarring and calcification of the valve, causing it to cease normal function. The scarring and calcification create a funnel-shaped opening between the left atrium and left ventricle.

The mitral stenosis murmur starts with an opening snap (OS) after A_2 and isovolumic relaxation (♦73____); this OS is an important diagnostic feature of mitral stenosis. The murmur is produced by rapid, turbulent blood flow through a rigid, narrowed mitral valve opening. Turbulence increases just before systole; this gives the murmur its characteristic presystolic crescendo.

Auscultatory area for normal pressure pulmonic valve murmur

1. Third intercostal space
2. Fourth intercostal space

PCG and ECG showing mitral stenosis murmur (atrial fibrillation)

PCG and ECG showing mitral stenosis murmur (normal sinus rhythm)

The more severe the stenosis, the longer the murmur's duration. In severe mitral stenosis, the murmur is holo-diastolic; in moderate stenosis, it appears in early and late diastole. The murmur ends with a loud M_1, which implies that the valve leaflets are mobile; the M_1 is often palpable. If the valve is calcified, S_1 is soft and an OS is not heard.

Mitral stenosis is sometimes associated with mitral regurgitation, so a systolic murmur may be heard as well. If mitral stenosis has caused pulmonary hypertension and right ventricular failure, tricuspid regurgitation may be the dominant murmur heard.

SOUND CHARACTERISTICS

The mitral stenosis murmur is usually heard best near the heart's apex over the mitral area. Its intensity and duration are variable. It has a low pitch heard best with the bell of the stethoscope and a rumbling quality that has been compared to thunder. The timing of a mitral stenosis murmur is diastolic: It begins after A_2 with an OS and ends with a loud M_1. (♦74____) However, stenosis severity affects the murmur's duration. In the ECG waveform, the murmur begins just after the T wave and ends during the QRS complex. It has a crescendo-decrescendo configuration. In patients with normal sinus rhythm, the presystolic component has a crescendo configuration. (♦75____)

ENHANCEMENT TECHNIQUES

The mitral stenosis murmur is heard best with the patient in a partial left lateral recumbent position. It can be intensified by maneuvers that increase cardiac output, such as having the patient exercise for a few minutes, raise his legs from a recumbent position, or cough several times.

Tricuspid stenosis murmurs

Tricuspid stenosis rarely occurs as an isolated defect; it's almost always associated with mitral valve defects. The tricuspid stenosis murmur begins shortly after a normal S_2 and is introduced by an OS that can be seen on a phonocardiogram (PCG) but that is seldom heard. (♦76____)

SOUND CHARACTERISTICS

The tricuspid stenosis murmur is usually heard best over the tricuspid area. Its usually soft intensity increases during inspiration and fades or disappears during expiration.

Area producing mitral stenosis murmur

Stenotic mitral valve

Auscultatory area for mitral stenosis murmur

Mitral area

Area producing tricuspid stenosis murmur

Stenotic tricuspid valve

PCG and ECG showing tricuspid stenosis murmur

Auscultatory area for tricuspid stenosis murmur

Tricuspid area

The murmur's duration is variable. It has a low pitch heard best with the bell of the stethoscope while the patient is in the partial left lateral recumbent position. The murmur has a rumbling quality. Its timing is mid- to late diastolic: It ends just before S_1. An OS may be heard. In the ECG waveform, the murmur begins just after the T wave and ends just before the QRS complex. In patients with normal sinus rhythm, it has a late diastolic crescendo or crescendo-decrescendo configuration. (♦77___)

AUSCULTATION TIP The tricuspid stenosis murmur can be differentiated from the mitral stenosis murmur because the murmur intensifies with inspiration while the mitral stenosis murmur doesn't.

◤ POSTTEST

1. How is the sound of a diastolic murmur produced?
2. Describe the characteristics of an early diastolic aortic regurgitation murmur.
3. How can an early diastolic aortic regurgitation murmur be enhanced?
4. Describe the characteristics of an Austin Flint murmur.
5. Describe the characteristics of a Graham Steell murmur.

6. How is a Graham Steell murmur enhanced?

7. Describe the characteristics of a normal pressure pulmonic valve murmur.

8. How is a normal pressure pulmonic valve murmur enhanced?

9. How is the sound of a mitral stenosis murmur produced?

10. Describe the characteristics of a mitral stenosis murmur.

11. How is a mitral stenosis murmur enhanced?

12. Describe the characteristics of a tricuspid stenosis murmur.

19

Continuous murmurs

▶️ *PRETEST*

1. How is the sound of a continuous murmur produced?
2. What is a cervical venous hum?
3. Why do the sounds of a patent ductus arteriosus (PDA) murmur change with age?
4. How can you differentiate between a PDA murmur and cervical venous hum murmur?

Two causes

Continuous murmurs are generated by rapid blood flow through arteries or veins or by shunting. Shunting occurs when an abnormal communication is created between the high-pressure arterial system and the low-pressure venous system. The murmurs begin in systole and persist, without interruption, through S_2 into diastole. Because these murmurs end late in diastole, they are continuous throughout the cardiac cycle.

Area producing cervical venous hum murmur

1. Internal jugular vein
2. Trachea

Cervical venous hum murmurs

The most common continuous murmur is the normal cervical venous hum, caused by rapid downward blood flow through the jugular veins in the lower part of the neck. (♦78____) The cervical venous hum is present in most individuals, but it's more pronounced in patients with hyperkinetic circulatory states, such as anemia, pregnancy, or thyrotoxicosis. The hum will disappear if the patient

PCG and ECG showing cervical venous hum murmur

performs Valsalva's maneuver, lies down, or has pressure applied over the jugular vein.

SOUND CHARACTERISTICS

The cervical venous hum murmur is heard best over the right supraclavicular fossa when the patient is sitting and his head is turned to the left. It has a faint intensity that increases during diastole. The murmur has a long duration: It lasts throughout the cardiac cycle. Its high pitch is heard best with the diaphragm of the stethoscope. Its quality is soft and its timing is continuous. The hum is louder between S_2 and S_1. (♦79____) The murmur has a plateau shape in systole and a crescendo-decrescendo configuration in diastole.

Auscultatory area for cervical venous hum murmur

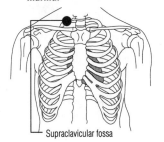

Supraclavicular fossa

Patent ductus arteriosus murmurs

The patent ductus arteriosus (PDA) murmur is the prototype of continuous murmurs. (♦80____) Normally, the ductus is open during fetal life and closes shortly after birth. When the ductus remains open, abnormal blood flow, or shunting, occurs from the high-pressure aorta to the low-

PCG and ECG showing patent ductus arteriosus murmur

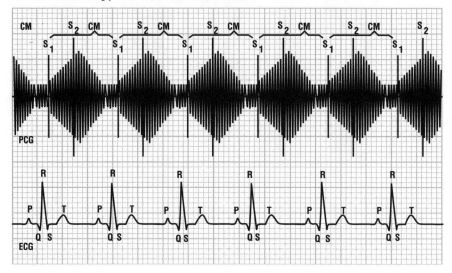

Area producing patent ductus arteriosus murmur

— Patent ductus arteriosus

Auscultatory area for patent ductus arteriosus murmur

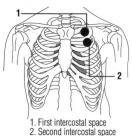

1. First intercostal space
2. Second intercostal space

pressure pulmonary artery. The PDA murmur extends into diastole. A thrill may be palpable in a loud PDA murmur.

SOUND CHARACTERISTICS

The PDA murmur is heard best over the entire left first and second intercostal spaces. Its intensity is faint when the murmur is limited to this area. If the murmur is loud, the systolic component may be heard along the left sternal border and sometimes over the mitral area. A loud PDA murmur may radiate to the back between the scapulae. The PDA murmur has a long duration. Its intensity is variable, roughly correlating with the ductus size; typically, the murmur reaches maximum intensity late in systole and then fades during diastole.

The PDA murmur has a high pitch heard equally well with the bell or diaphragm of the stethoscope. It has a rough, machinery-like quality, and its timing is continuous. It begins with, or shortly after, a normal S_1 and disappears just before the next S_1. Because the murmur peaks in late systole, S_2 may be difficult to hear. S_2 may be paradoxically split if left ventricular ejection time is prolonged. An S_3 may be heard over the mitral area. (◆81____) The murmur has a crescendo-decrescendo configuration.

ENHANCEMENT TECHNIQUES

Exercise can increase the intensity and duration of a PDA murmur.

Differentiating PDA murmurs from cervical venous hum murmurs

To differentiate these two murmurs, remember that the hum is loudest above the clavicle, is usually heard better on the right, and can be obliterated by pressing on the jugular vein or placing the patient in a supine position. The venous hum is truly continuous and is usually louder during diastole.

◤ *POSTTEST*

1. How is the sound of a continuous murmur produced?
2. What causes a cervical venous hum?
3. Describe the characteristics of a cervical venous hum murmur.
4. Describe the characteristics of a PDA murmur.
5. How can a PDA murmur be enhanced?
6. How can you differentiate between a PDA murmur and a cervical venous hum murmur?

20

Other auscultatory sounds

▶️ PRETEST

1. What are the four types of prosthetic valves?
2. What are the similarities and differences of the sounds produced by the four types of aortic prosthetic valves?
3. How do you know if an aortic prosthetic valve is malfunctioning?
4. What are the similarities and differences of the sounds produced by the four types of mitral prosthetic valves?
5. How do you know if a mitral prosthetic valve is malfunctioning?
6. What produces a pericardial friction rub?
7. What is mediastinal crunch?

Prosthetic valve sounds and murmurs

Prosthetic heart valves are used to replace malfunctioning human valves. The aortic and mitral valves are the ones most commonly replaced. The tricuspid valve is replaced occasionally; the pulmonic valve, rarely. The following discussion will focus on the aortic and mitral valves.

Four types of prosthetic valves are used to replace human valves: the ball-in-cage, the tilting-disk, the bileaflet, and the porcine valves. (See *Ball-in-cage valve* and *Tilting-disk valve,* page 172; *Bileaflet valve,* page 173; and *Porcine valve,* page 174.)

When a prosthetic valve is surgically placed in the aortic orifice, it's positioned so that it opens during systole and closes at the beginning of diastole. However, when a prosthetic valve is surgically placed in the mitral orifice, it's positioned so that it closes at the beginning of systole and opens during diastole.

An aortic prosthetic valve will not change a normal S_1, and a mitral prosthetic valve will not change a normal S_2. However, prosthetic valves do produce characteristic auscultatory sounds and murmurs. For example, some prostheses produce opening clicks, and all prostheses, regardless of type or position, produce closing clicks. The ball-in-cage valve produces the loudest sounds.

Typically, any disappearance or muffling of previously heard prosthetic valve sounds or murmurs, or the development of a new murmur in a patient with a prosthetic valve, indicates possible prosthetic valve dysfunction.

All prosthetic valves in the aortic and mitral positions are associated with a soft early systolic or midsystolic ejection murmur. This murmur is heard best over the tricuspid, mitral, and aortic areas and is similar to the mild aortic stenosis murmur.

Some prosthetic valves in the mitral position produce a short, soft, rumbling early diastolic murmur, which is very similar to the mitral stenosis murmur except that it's brief and a presystolic component isn't heard. This murmur is heard best near the heart's apex over the mitral area while the patient is in the partial left lateral recumbent position.

Aortic prosthetic valves

Distinctive sounds and murmurs are associated with the various types of prostheses used in aortic valve replacement. (♦82____)

Aortic ball-in-cage valve
A normally functioning aortic ball-in-cage valve prosthesis doesn't change the normal S_1 characteristics. S_1 is followed by an aortic opening click that's louder than S_1; it's sharp, high-pitched, and has a crisp quality. An aortic closing click replaces A_2. Although the aortic ball-in-cage valve prosthesis is no longer inserted, patients with this type of prosthesis may still be seen.

SOUND CHARACTERISTICS
The murmur generated by an aortic ball-in-cage valve prosthesis is usually heard best near the apex over the mitral and aortic areas and along the left sternal border. Its intensity is usually loud and easy to hear, and its duration is variable. It has a medium pitch heard best with the di-

Auscultatory area for aortic and mitral prosthetic valve murmurs with systolic ejection murmur

1. Aortic area
2. Tricuspid area
3. Mitral area

Auscultatory area for mitral prosthetic valve murmur with early diastolic murmur

Mitral area

Ball-in-cage valve

PCG showing aortic ball-in-cage valve murmur

aphragm of the stethoscope. The murmur has a crunchy, harsh quality. Its timing is midsystolic. The interval between the aortic closing click and P_2 is similar to the normal $A_2 - P_2$ interval, and it normally widens during inspiration. The murmur has a crescendo-decrescendo configuration.

Detecting a malfunctioning aortic ball-in-cage valve

Dysfunction of an aortic ball-in-cage valve prosthesis commonly causes the aortic opening click to become soft or absent; the aortic closing click may be absent too. A diastolic murmur and a long systolic ejection murmur (SEM) may appear.

Aortic tilting-disk valve

S_1 is unchanged with a normally functioning aortic tilting-disk valve prosthesis. An aortic opening click may be heard, and the interval between the aortic closing click and P_2 is normal. The aortic closing click isn't as loud as the click heard with a ball-in-cage prosthesis.

PCG showing aortic tilting-disk valve murmur

Tilting-disk valve

Dotted line indicates that valve opening may or may not be heard.

SOUND CHARACTERISTICS
The murmur generated by an aortic tilting-disk valve prosthesis is usually heard best near the apex over the mitral and aortic areas and along the left sternal border. Its intensity is usually soft (grade $\%$), and its duration is short. It has a medium pitch heard best with the diaphragm of the stethoscope. The murmur has a rough or harsh quality. Its timing is systolic. The interval between the aortic closing click and P_2 is similar to the normal $A_2 - P_2$ interval, and it widens during inspiration. The murmur has a crescendo-decrescendo configuration.

Detecting a malfunctioning aortic tilting-disk valve

Dysfunction of an aortic tilting-disk valve prosthesis commonly causes some or all of the following changes: The aortic closing click may be absent, a diastolic murmur may be heard, a murmur that extends into the latter half of diastole may appear, or a longer SEM may appear.

Aortic bileaflet valve

S_1 is normal with a normally functioning aortic bileaflet valve prosthesis. The aortic opening click may be inaudible, but the closing click is loud and distinct.

SOUND CHARACTERISTICS
The murmur generated by an aortic bileaflet valve prosthesis is usually heard best near the apex over the mitral and aortic areas and along the left sternal border. Its intensity is usually soft (grade $\%$), and its duration is short. It has a medium pitch heard best with the diaphragm of the stethoscope. The murmur has a rough or harsh quality, and its timing is systolic. The interval between the aortic closing click and P_2 is similar to the normal $A_2 - P_2$ interval, and it widens during inspiration. The murmur has a crescendo-decrescendo configuration.

PCG showing aortic bileaflet valve murmur

Bileaflet valve

PCG

S_1

SM

P_2

Valve opens

Valve closes

Porcine valve

PCG showing aortic porcine valve murmur

Dotted line indicates that valve opening may or may not be heard.

Detecting a malfunctioning aortic bileaflet valve

Dysfunction of the aortic bileaflet valve prosthesis may cause the aortic closing click to disappear, a diastolic murmur to appear, or both. A longer SEM also may appear.

Aortic porcine valve

S_2 is normal with a normally functioning aortic porcine valve prosthesis. The aortic opening click is soft or inaudible.

SOUND CHARACTERISTICS

The murmur generated by an aortic porcine valve prosthesis is usually heard best near the apex over the mitral and aortic areas and along the left sternal border. Its intensity is usually soft (grade $\frac{2}{6}$), and its duration is short. It has a medium pitch heard best with the diaphragm of the stethoscope. The murmur has a rough or harsh quality, and its timing is systolic. The interval between the aortic closing click and P_2 is similar to the normal $A_2 - P_2$ interval, and it widens during inspiration. The murmur has a crescendo-decrescendo configuration.

Detecting a malfunctioning aortic porcine valve

Dysfunction of an aortic porcine valve prosthesis may cause the aortic closing click to be diminished, a diastolic murmur to appear, or both. A longer SEM also may appear.

Mitral prosthetic valves

Distinctive sounds and murmurs are associated with the various types of prostheses used in mitral valve replacement. (♦83_____)

PCG showing mitral ball-in-cage valve murmur

Parentheses around S₁ indicate that S₁ will not be heard because valve closure is louder.

Mitral ball-in-cage valve

The mitral closing click replaces M_1 with a normally functioning mitral ball-in-cage valve prosthesis. Some patients with this type of prosthetic valve have middiastolic clicks or short, soft (grade ⅖), rumbling diastolic murmurs that are heard best near the apex over the mitral area with the patient in a partial left lateral recumbent position.

SOUND CHARACTERISTICS
When the systolic murmur generated by a mitral ball-in-cage valve prosthesis is audible, it's usually heard best near the apex over the mitral or tricuspid area. Its intensity is usually soft, and its duration is short. It has a medium pitch heard best with the diaphragm of the stethoscope. The murmur has a harsh quality, and its timing is systolic. A mitral opening click follows a normal S_2. The murmur has a crescendo-decrescendo configuration.

Detecting a malfunctioning mitral ball-in-cage valve
Dysfunction of a mitral ball-in-cage valve prosthesis may cause some or all of the following changes: The sounds normally associated with the valve may vary in intensity in a patient with normal sinus rhythm; a short interval between A_2 and the mitral opening click may occur, indicating high left atrial pressure; a holosystolic murmur may occur, indicating mitral regurgitation; or the intensity and duration of the diastolic murmur may change, indicating mitral obstruction.

Mitral tilting-disk valve

A normally functioning mitral tilting-disk valve prosthesis replaces M_1, with a mitral closing click. This closing click is always distinctly audible and high-pitched; its max-

PCG showing mitral tilting-disk valve murmur

Dotted line indicates that valve opening may or may not be heard.
Parentheses around S₁ indicate that S₁ will not be heard because valve closure is louder.

imum intensity is located near the apex over the mitral area. A mitral opening click may follow a normal S_2.

SOUND CHARACTERISTICS
The systolic murmur generated by a mitral tilting-disk valve prosthesis is usually heard best near the apex over the mitral area or, occasionally, over the tricuspid area. Its intensity is usually soft (grade ⅔). The murmur has a short duration and a high pitch heard best with the diaphragm of the stethoscope. It has a harsh quality and systolic timing. The murmur has a crescendo-decrescendo configuration.

Detecting a malfunctioning mitral tilting-disk valve
Dysfunction of a mitral tilting-disk valve prosthesis may cause some or all of the following changes: The mitral closing click may be absent, a new diastolic murmur may develop, a previously auscultated diastolic murmur may intensify, or a holosystolic mitral regurgitation murmur may appear.

Mitral bileaflet valve
A normally functioning mitral bileaflet valve prosthesis replaces M_1 with a mitral closing click that is loud and high-pitched. The mitral opening click, however, may be inaudible. If it's audible, it follows a normal S_2. In about 50% of patients with a mitral bileaflet valve prosthesis, a short middiastolic rumble occurs; this rumble is heard best near the apex over the mitral area.

SOUND CHARACTERISTICS
The systolic murmur generated by a mitral bileaflet valve prosthesis is usually heard best near the apex over the mitral area or, occasionally, over the tricuspid area. Its intensity is usually soft (grade ⅔), and its duration is short.

PCG showing mitral bileaflet valve murmur

Parentheses around S_1 indicate that S_1 will not be heard because valve closure is louder.

It has a high pitch heard best with the diaphragm of the stethoscope. The murmur has a harsh quality and its timing is systolic. The mitral opening click, though rarely heard, follows a normal S_2. The murmur has a crescendo-decrescendo configuration.

Detecting a malfunctioning mitral bileaflet valve
Dysfunction of a mitral bileaflet valve prosthesis may cause a holosystolic murmur, a new diastolic murmur, or both to appear.

Mitral porcine valve
A normally functioning mitral porcine valve prosthesis generates a mitral closing click that is heard over the mitral area and that sounds like a normal M_1. A mitral opening click after a normal S_2 is heard in about 50% of patients with this type of valve.

SOUND CHARACTERISTICS
The systolic murmur generated by a mitral porcine valve prosthesis has a crescendo-decrescendo configuration. The murmur is usually heard best near the apex over the

PCG showing mitral porcine valve murmur

Auscultatory area for pericardial friction rub

1. Tricuspid area
2. Xyphoid area

mitral area. Its intensity is usually soft (grade ⅖ to ⅜), and its duration is short. It has a medium pitch heard best with the diaphragm of the stethoscope and a harsh quality. Its timing is systolic. ·

Detecting a malfunctioning mitral porcine valve
Dysfunction of a mitral porcine valve prosthesis may cause a holosystolic mitral regurgitation murmur, a diastolic rumble associated with mitral stenosis, or both to appear.

Pericardial friction rubs

When inflamed pericardial surfaces rub together, they produce characteristic high-pitched friction noises known as pericardial friction rubs. (♦84____) These rubs are a classic sign of pericarditis (inflammation of the pericardium, the sac surrounding the heart), which can be caused by viral or bacterial infections, radiation therapy to the chest, or cardiac trauma. Pericardial friction rubs may also be heard after a pericardiotomy and for a few hours to a few days after a myocardial infarction.

SOUND CHARACTERISTICS
A pericardial friction rub is usually heard best, and is sometimes palpable, over the tricuspid and xyphoid areas. It's usually loud and may get louder during inspiration. The rub has a high pitch heard best with the diaphragm of the stethoscope, and it has a grating or scratchy quality. It's usually heard during each cardiac cycle. It has a systolic component and an early and late diastolic component. (♦85____) The diastolic component may last for only a few hours.

⊚ **AUSCULTATION TIP** To differentiate a pericardial friction rub from a pleural friction rub, have the patient hold his breath. When he does so, a pericardial friction rub will persist, but a pleural friction rub will become inaudible.

Mediastinal crunch

Heart movements can displace air that's present in the mediastinum; this displacement produces crunchy noises—known as mediastinal crunch—which may occur randomly or in a consistent pattern. (♦86____) Patients with mediastinal crunch commonly have subcutaneous emphysema (air trapped beneath the skin). You can assess for this condition by palpating for crepitation in the neck.

SOUND CHARACTERISTICS

The noises produced by mediastinal crunch are usually heard best near the apex over the mitral area and along the left sternal border with the patient in the partial left lateral recumbent position. The noises have a crunching quality, which may become louder during inspiration. (♦87____)

Auscultatory area for mediastinal crunch

1. Left sternal border
2. Mitral area

POSTTEST

1. Which two valves are most commonly replaced?
2. What are the four types of prosthetic valves?
3. Describe the characteristics of an aortic ball-in-cage valve murmur.
4. What changes in sounds can you expect if an aortic ball-in-cage valve malfunctions?
5. Describe the characteristics of an aortic tilting-disk murmur.
6. What changes in sounds can you expect if an aortic tilting-disk valve malfunctions?
7. Describe the characteristics of an aortic bileaflet valve murmur.
8. What changes in sounds can you expect if an aortic bileaflet valve malfunctions?
9. Describe the characteristics of an aortic porcine valve murmur.
10. What changes in sounds can you expect if an aortic porcine valve malfunctions?
11. Describe the characteristics of a mitral ball-in-cage valve murmur.
12. What changes in sounds can you expect if a mitral ball-in-cage valve malfunctions?
13. Describe the characteristics of a mitral tilting-disk murmur.
14. What changes in sounds can you expect if a mitral tilting-disk valve malfunctions?
15. Describe the characteristics of a mitral bileaflet valve murmur.
16. What changes in sounds can you expect if a mitral bileaflet valve malfunctions?
17. Describe the characteristics of a mitral porcine valve murmur.

18. What changes in sounds can you expect if a mitral porcine valve malfunctions?
19. What causes a pericardial friction rub?
20. Describe the characteristics of a pericardial friction rub.
21. How can you differentiate between a pericardial and a pleural friction rub?
22. What is mediastinal crunch?
23. Describe the characteristics of mediastinal crunch.

Appendix: Auscultation findings for common disorders

Posttest answers

Selected references

Glossary

Index

Appendix: Auscultation findings for common disorders

The following is a compilation of various cardiac and pulmonary disorders along with associated auscultation findings. The patient may not present with every assessment finding listed for each disorder.

Disorder	Abnormal breath sounds	Abnormal heart sounds
Aortic prosthetic valve		• Systolic murmur • Aortic opening click • Aortic closing click • Interval between aortic closing click and P_2 that widens during inspiration
Aortic regurgitation		• Early diastolic murmur often with midsystolic murmur • Diminished A_2 • Early ejection click • Paradoxical S_2 split • S_3–S_4 gallop • Soft S_1
Aortic valvular stenosis	• Inspiratory and expiratory crackles over the posterior lung bases associated with heart failure	• Midsystolic murmur • Paradoxical S_2 split • Delayed A_2 and shortened A_2–P_2 interval • Aortic ejection sound • Systolic ejection sound if not severely stenotic
Asbestosis	• Loud, continuous, high-pitched, sequential wheezes	
Asthma	• Diminished breath sounds • Musical, high-pitched expiratory polyphonic wheezes	

Disorder	Abnormal breath sounds	Abnormal heart sounds
Asthma (*continued*)	• With status asthmaticus, loud and continuous random monophonic wheezes heard, along with prolonged expiration and possible silent chest	
Atelectasis	• High-pitched, hollow, tubular bronchial breath sounds • Late inspiratory crackles • Bronchophony • Egophony • Whispered pectoriloquy • I:E ratio 1:1	
Atrial septal defect		• Wide fixed S_2 split • Pulmonic ejection sound
Bronchial stenosis	• Loud, continuous, low pitched, fixed, monophonic wheezes which may disappear when in supine position or turning side to side	
Bronchiectasis	• Profuse, low-pitched crackles heard during mid-inspiration	
Chronic bronchitis	• Scanty, low-pitched, early inspiratory crackles not affected by patient's position • Loud, musical, high-pitched, expiratory polyphonic wheezes	
Chronic obstructive pulmonary disease	• Diminished, low-pitched breath sounds • Wheezes • Inaudible bronchophony, egophony, and whispered pectoriloquy	

(continued)

Disorder	Abnormal breath sounds	Abnormal heart sounds
Fibrosing alveolitis	• Loud, continuous, high-pitched, sequential wheezes	
Hypertrophic obstructive cardiomyopathy	• Inspiratory and expiratory crackles over the posterior lung bases associated with heart failure	• Midsystolic murmur that becomes louder with Valsalva's maneuver • Paradoxical S_2 split • Abnormal S_3 and S_4
Interstitial pulmonary fibrosis	• High-pitched bronchial breath sounds heard over lower lung regions that are audible through inspiration and expiration • Late inspiratory fine crackles not affected by coughing but may disappear with position change, deep inhalation, or holding of breath • Loud, high-pitched sequential wheezes of continuous duration	
Laryngeal spasm	• Stridor heard during inspiration	
Malfunctioning aortic prosthetic valve	• Inspiratory and expiratory crackles over the posterior lung bases associated with heart failure	• Long systolic ejection murmur • Absent or softened aortic opening click • Absent or diminished aortic closing click • Diastolic murmur
Malfunctioning mitral prosthetic valve	• Inspiratory and expiratory crackles over the posterior lung bases associated with heart failure	• Holosystolic murmur • New diastolic murmur or change in intensity or duration of existing one • Diastolic rumble • Absent mitral closing click

Disorder	Abnormal breath sounds	Abnormal heart sounds
Mitral prosthetic valve		• Systolic murmur • Mitral closing click • Mitral opening click depending on valve type • Diastolic murmur — soft and short
Mitral regurgitation	• Inspiratory and expiratory crackles over the posterior lung bases associated with heart failure	• Holosystolic murmur • Decreased S_1 intensity • S_2 intensity increased • Accented P_2 • S_3 and S_4 gallop • Persistent A_2–P_2 splitting during expiration
Mitral stenosis		• With moderate stenosis, early and late diastolic murmur • In severe stenosis, possibly holodiastolic murmur • Loud M_1 • Intensified S_1 except with a calcified valve, which produces a soft S_1 • Split S_2 • Opening snap except with a calcified valve • S_3 gallop
Mitral valve prolapse		• Late systolic or holosystolic murmur • Non-ejection midsystolic click that's variable in intensity and timing • Precordial honk
Myocardial infarction	• Inspiratory and expiratory crackles over the posterior lung bases associated with heart failure	• A_2 intensity diminished • Abnormal S_4

(continued)

Disorder	Abnormal breath sounds	Abnormal heart sounds
Patent ductus arteriosus		• Continuous murmur reaching maximum intensity during late systole • Paradoxical S_2 split • S_3
Pericarditis		• Pericardial friction rub, which has both a systolic and diastolic component
Pleural effusion	• Absent or diminished low-pitched breath sounds • Occasionally loud bronchial breath sounds • Normal breath sounds on contralateral side • Bronchophony, egophony, and whispered pectoriloquy at upper border of pleural effusion	
Pneumonia	• High-pitched, tubular bronchial breath sounds heard over right posterior mid-lung field audible during inspiration and expiration • Bronchophony • Egophony • Whispered pectoriloquy • Late inspiratory crackles not affected by coughing or position changes • I:E ratio 1:2	
Pneumothorax	• Absent or diminished low-pitched breath sounds • Inaudible bronchophony, egophony, and whispered pectoriloquy • Normal breath sounds heard on contralateral side	

Disorder	Abnormal breath sounds	Abnormal heart sounds
Pulmonary edema	• Inspiratory and expiratory crackles over the posterior lung bases; as pulmonary edema worsens, crackles more profuse and heard during late inspiration • Wheezes	• S_3 or S_4
Pulmonic regurgitation		• Early diastolic murmur intensified during inspiration • Loud P_2
Pulmonic valve stenosis		• Midsystolic murmur • Systolic ejection click • P_2 absent or diminished • Normal or widened S_2 split • S_4
Supravalvular aortic stenosis		• Midsystolic murmur • Normal S_2 split • No aortic ejection sound
Tricuspid stenosis		• Mid-to-late diastolic murmur, which increases during inspiration and fades during expiration • Normal S_2 or may be split during inspiration • Opening snap seldom heard
Ventricular septal defect		• Persistent A_2–P_2 splitting during expiration • Abnormal S_3 • Pulmonic ejection sound
Whooping cough	• Stridor	

Posttest answers

Breath sounds

1 The respiratory system and auscultation

1. The respiratory system's primary function is the exchange of oxygen (O_2) and carbon dioxide (CO_2) between the alveoli and the pulmonary circulation.
2. The upper airway consists of the nasal cavities and the pharynx.
3. The pharynx is divided into three sections: the nasopharynx, the oropharynx, and the hypopharynx.
4. The lower airway is called the tracheobronchial tree. It begins at the larynx and ends at the distal bronchioles, which open into the alveoli.
5. Anteriorly, the trachea begins just below the larynx and is located within the thoracic cavity, beneath the upper two-thirds of the sternum. Posteriorly, it begins at the level of the sixth cervical or first thoracic vertebra and extends to approximately the fifth thoracic vertebra.
6. The mainstem bronchi enter the lungs at the hila, where the lung tissue attaches to the mediastinum. The bronchi course downward and immediately divide into lobar bronchi, which subdivide into segmental bronchi. The airways continue to systematically branch, narrow, shorten, and increase in number toward the lung periphery. They divide approximately 25 times before ultimately opening into the terminal, or respiratory, bronchioles. The terminal bronchioles, which have a few alveoli budding from their walls, branch into the alveolar ducts, which are completely lined with alveoli.
7. Anatomic dead space is the approximately 150 cc of air that remain in the conducting airways during each breath. This air is not involved in O_2–CO_2 exchange.
8. The mucous and bronchial glands located in the bronchial walls secrete a serous mucus blanket onto the inside airway walls. This secreted mucus forms a thin, sticky layer that lies on top of ciliated columnar epithelial cells, which line nearly all of the respiratory tract between the larynx and the terminal bronchioles. The mucus layer traps foreign particles in the inspired air before they can enter the lungs. The cilia move in a wavelike motion, propelling the sticky mucus layer toward the pharynx. Together, the mucus layer and cilia protect the

lungs, acting as a major defense mechanism against inhaled particles.

9. Each lung is divided into lobes. The right lung has three lobes: the upper, middle, and lower. The left lung has only an upper and a lower lobe.

10. The lung's apex (superior aspect) is located near the clavicle, and its base (inferior aspect) is located near the diaphragm.

11. Alveoli contain three cell types. Type 1, the largest, is the lining cell and accounts for 95% of the alveolar surface area. The type II cell is believed to produce surfactant, a mixture of phospholipids. The macrophage, the third cell type, acts as a phagocytic defense mechanism against infection.

12. Surfactant is a mixture of phospholipids found in the fluid layer that covers the alveolar surface. The surfactant mixes with pulmonary fluids and maintains alveolar stability by lowering the alveolar surface tension, thus preventing the air filled alveoli from collapsing at low volumes from the weight of the capillary blood.

13. The parasympathetic nervous system in the larynx, trachea, and bronchi includes vagal nerve fibers and irritant receptors mediated by the neurotransmitter acetylcholine. Parasympathetic stimulation precipitates bronchoconstriction, coughing, and mucus discharge from the bronchial glands. Irritant receptors within the airways are believed to be responsible for increasing ventilation and precipitating coughing.

   Sympathetic innervation of the lower airways usually arises from the thoracic nerves T1 through T5 and is mediated by the postganglionic hormone transmitter norepinephrine. Sympathetic stimulation of adrenergic beta$_2$-receptors throughout the lower airways facilitates smooth muscle relaxation, resulting in bronchodilation.

14. The pulmonary circulation begins as the pulmonary artery leaves the right ventricle. The pulmonary artery divides into segmental arteries, which subdivide, ending in the pulmonary capillary bed surrounding the alveoli. The capillaries then join to form venules, which converge to form veins, then pulmonary veins. The pulmonary veins end in the left atrium.

15. The bronchial circulation usually originates in the aorta and branches along the bronchi to provide oxygen and nutrients to the lung tissue and to clear meta-

bolic wastes from the airways and other lung tissues. Oxygenated blood is pumped from the aorta to the tracheobronchial tree and travels through arterioles along the airways. Deoxygenated blood from the bronchial circulation is returned to the left atrium, accounting for the normal 2% to 3% right-to-left shunt.

16. The chest wall's inner surface and the lungs' outer surfaces are joined by thin, membranous tissues called the pleurae. The parietal pleura covers the chest wall's inner surface, and the visceral pleura covers the lungs' outer surfaces.

17. The thorax is the bony structure that protects the vital organs (the heart and lungs) and permits chest expansion during inspiration.

18. The diaphragm, the primary muscle of respiration, consists of two dome-shaped hemidiaphragms that are attached to the lower edge of the rib cage. The diaphragm forms the inferior "floor" of the thorax. During inspiration, the diaphragm flattens and descends toward the abdomen. During expiration, it relaxes and ascends to its resting, dome-shaped configuration.

19. The external intercostal muscles, located between the ribs and innervated by the intercostal nerves, contract during inspiration to stabilize, elevate, and expand the rib cage.

20. The accessory muscles of respiration — the sternocleidomastoid, scalene, trapezius, and rhomboid muscles — are involved in labored or forceful breathing. The sternocleidomastoid muscle elevates the sternum, increasing the anterior-to-posterior chest diameter. The scalene muscles elevate and fix the first two ribs. The trapezius and rhomboid muscles are activated during respiration but probably have no effect on forceful inspiration. The contraction of external intercostal muscles may also be obvious in extremely labored breathing.

21. During inspiration, the diaphragm and external intercostal muscles are activated. Diaphragmatic contraction flattens the domed diaphragm and expands the lower rib cage, forcing the abdominal contents downward and out, thus increasing the longitudinal lung size. External intercostal muscle contraction stabilizes the rib cage and moves it outward and upward. The posterior cricoarytenoid muscle contracts to open the glottis. As the thorax expands, intrapleural pres-

sures become subatmospheric, resulting in lung expansion and decreased intrapulmonary pressures. Inspired air flows from higher atmospheric pressure into the airways. At the end of inspiration, diaphragmatic movement declines and the air inflow gradually slows.

During expiration, the thorax and the elastic recoil force of the lungs return to their resting positions, increasing intrapleural pressures. This increased pressure forces air to flow out of the lower and upper airways. At the end of expiration, during quiet breathing, all muscles are relaxed and the diaphragm has returned to its resting position.

22. During normal breathing in the upright position, air movement (ventilation) is greatest in the lung bases or dependent lung regions. Because of the pull of gravity, the alveoli in the lung bases collapse to a smaller size during expiration than do the alveoli in the lung apices. During inspiration, the alveoli in the lung bases open more easily, causing ventilation in the bases to be greater than in the apices.

Blood perfusion in the lungs is also gravity-dependent; the dependent lung regions receive a larger proportion of the cardiac output than the nondependent regions.

23. Postural changes affect the distribution of ventilation and blood flow throughout the lungs. In the supine position, the apices and bases receive equal amounts of air and blood flow. In the lateral position, dependent lung regions receive more air and blood flow than nondependent regions.

24. The tracheobronchial tree's dimensions and shape affect the airflow pattern as follows: During inspiration, air velocity and the airflow rate decrease as the cross-sectional airway area increases. Consequently, the larger airways conduct the same volume of air as do the more numerous smaller airways. This means that inspired air travels 100 times faster in the trachea than it does in the terminal bronchi. Beyond the terminal bronchi, the forward movement of air is minimal. In the terminal bronchioles, diffusion is the primary method of air movement.

25. The lung apices extend approximately ¼″ to 1½″ (2 to 4 cm) above the clavicles. The trachea bifurcates at the level of the sternal angle, the junction between the manubrium and the body of the sternum. The

ribs and intercostal spaces provide precise horizontal landmarks to describe the location of breath sounds; the second rib and second intercostal space serve as reference points.

Vertical landmark lines on the anterior chest wall surface include the midclavicular lines and the midsternal line. The right and left midclavicular lines extend downward from the center of each clavicle. The midsternal line bisects the sternum. The right lung base crosses the sixth rib at the right midclavicular line, and the left lung base crosses the seventh rib at the left midclavicular line.

26. The anterior axillary line extends downward from the anterior axillary fold, the midaxillary line extends downward from the apex of the axilla, and the posterior axillary line extends downward from the posterior axillary fold.

27. Bony structures underlying the posterior chest wall surface also provide landmarks to locate breath sounds. The scapulae's inferior borders, located at about the same level as the seventh rib, serve as reference points. The numbered thoracic vertebrae provide horizontal landmarks. Landmark lines on the posterior chest wall surface provide vertical reference points. The midscapular lines extend downward from the inferior angle of each scapula, and the vertebral line extends downward over the vertebrae.

28. The diaphragm of the stethoscope attenuates low-pitched sound frequencies, so it's used to listen for high-pitched breath sounds; the bell attenuates high-pitched sound frequencies, so it is used to listen for low-pitched breath sounds.

29. During auscultation, press the diaphragm of the stethoscope firmly against the patient's chest wall over the intercostal spaces. Try not to listen directly over bone; never listen through clothing, which impedes or alters sound transmission.

30. If the patient is alert and healthy, begin auscultation with the patient sitting upright and leaning slightly forward with his hands grasping his elbows to separate the scapulae. Position yourself behind the patient. Ask the patient to breathe through an open mouth, slightly deeper and faster than usual, through several respiratory cycles. Place the diaphragm of the stethoscope over the left lung apex, and listen for at least one complete respiratory cycle. Then move the

diaphragm to the same site over the right lung. Compare the breath sounds heard over these same locations. Continue in this manner, making contralateral comparisons at each auscultatory site.

2 Introduction to breath sounds

1. Breath sounds are produced by airflow patterns, by associated pressure changes within the airways, and by solid tissue vibrations.

2. Sounds heard over the trachea and large airways are characterized as loud and tubular (hollow) with a long expiratory phase. These sounds are thought to reflect the turbulent airflow patterns in the first divisions of the large airways. Sounds heard over other chest wall areas are softer and have a shorter expiratory phase.

3. An airway's stability depends on the interaction among the elastic properties of the lung tissue, the intrapulmonary airways, and the pressures — both internal and external — exerted on the airways. During the respiratory cycle, a pressure gradient exists across the airway wall and between the trachea and alveoli. As the chest expands during inspiration, intrapleural pressure falls. At the same time, the lung's elastic recoil increases, exerting traction on airway walls. This traction increases the airways' diameter and decreases the resistance to airflow. The pressure gradient between the alveolar and atmospheric pressures increases; this drives air through the airways toward the alveoli.

4. Intrapleural pressure and alveolar elastic recoil pressures drive expiratory airflow. At the beginning of expiration, intrapleural pressure and the alveolar recoil force cause the alveolar pressures to rise and push the air through the airways and out through the mouth. Air pressures fall as the air flows through the airways from the alveoli to the mouth. A point is reached, particularly during forceful expiration, when intrapleural and intrapulmonary pressures are equal; this normally occurs in the segmental bronchi and is called the equal pressure point. Downstream from this point, pressures outside of the airways can compress and further narrow the airways, causing increased resistance to airflow.

5. Variations in airflow patterns are affected by the intricate network of branching airways, the various air-

way diameters, and the potential for irregular airway wall surfaces within the tracheobronchial tree.

6. During rapid, or turbulent, airflow, air molecules move randomly, colliding against airway walls and each other. They may move across or against the general direction of airflow. The colliding air molecules produce rapid pressure changes within the airway, and these rapid pressure changes produce sounds. Turbulent airflow occurs in the trachea, mainstem bronchi, and other larger airways.

7. As airflow is forced to change directions abruptly in the branching airways, the airstream separates into layers and moves at different velocities. The shearing force of high-velocity airstreams, along with slower airstreams, precipitates opposing circular airflows, or vortices. This airflow pattern generates sounds as the flow of air carries the vortices downstream.

8. In the terminal or small airways and respiratory bronchioles, airflow is slow and laminar. No abrupt changes in pressure or airway wall movements occur to generate sound. Consequently, air movement in these areas produces no sound.

9. Frequency, measured in hertz, refers to the number of vibrations occurring per unit of time. The term pitch is used to describe sound frequency. High-pitched sounds have higher frequencies; low-pitched sounds have lower frequencies. Intensity is the loudness or softness of the vibrations producing breath sounds. It can be measured electronically by recording amplitude. Intensity is affected by the type of vibrating structure producing the sound, the distance the sound travels, and the transmission pathway. The duration of the vibrations that produce breath sounds can be measured in milliseconds. However, the human ear perceives sounds during auscultation as long or short and as continuous or discontinuous.

10. Body structures or cavities that produce resonance will selectively transmit or amplify breath sounds that are similar in frequency and will absorb or dampen those with other frequencies. Breath sounds arising from the same location in the lung have a higher pitch when heard at the mouth or over the trachea than when heard over the chest wall. This change in pitch occurs because high-pitched breath sounds are absorbed as they are transmitted through the lungs and thorax.

11. Breath and voice sounds are normally damped when they are transmitted through air, fluid, and tissue. But when these sounds are transmitted sequentially through media with different acoustical properties, the sounds' vibrations are filtered and reflected at the interface of the different media. The amount of filtering that takes place depends on the media's impedance (resistance to sound transmission).

    When two media are matched according to acoustical properties, sound is transmitted effectively. For example, consolidated areas enhance the transmission of breath sounds to the chest wall. This happens because the consolidating substance, an inflammatory exudate, collects in alveoli, replacing air with dense lung tissue. Consequently, the fluid-filled, airless lung tissue and the chest wall are acoustically well matched, and breath sounds are transmitted more easily.

12. The transmission of breath and voice sounds through either air or fluid between inflated lung segments and the chest wall results in an impedance mismatch. The vibrations of the sounds are significantly filtered and reflected back to their source by the pleurae.

13. The tracheal and mainstem bronchi sounds, produced by turbulent airflow, are loud and can be heard throughout inspiration and expiration over the trachea and mainstem bronchi. Normal breath sounds heard over other chest wall areas are faint and can be heard throughout inspiration and at the beginning of expiration.

14. Many clinicians think bronchovesicular breath sounds represent a third classification of normal sounds. These sounds are heard over areas between the mainstem bronchi and the smaller airways; their pitch and duration are midway between those of tracheal and mainstem bronchi breath sounds and normal breath sounds heard over other chest wall areas. Bronchovesicular sounds are heard during inspiration and expiration for equal amounts of time.

15. Voice sounds auscultated over the chest wall are called bronchophony. In a healthy individual, bronchophony is similar to voice sounds heard through the neck. Voice sounds transmitted through the chest wall that have selectively amplified higher frequencies are called egophony. High-pitched whispered sounds transmitted through airless, consolidated lung tissue are called whispered pectoriloquy.

16. Adventitious sounds are added sounds that are heard with normal and abnormal breath sounds. They are divided into two classifications: crackles and wheezes.

17. Location, intensity, duration, and pitch are the four characteristics used to describe breath sounds.

18. Sound intensity is described subjectively, using such terms as loud, soft, absent, diminished, or distant.

19. Sound duration refers to the sound's timing within the respiratory cycle — that is, whether it's heard during inspiration, expiration, or both. Timing can be described as early, late, or throughout.

20. Sound pitch is usually described as high or low.

3 Breath sounds heard in healthy individuals

1. Normal breath sounds are broadly defined as breathing heard through the chest wall of a healthy individual.

2. Three variables affect the normal sounds heard during auscultation: the distance between the source of the sound and the chest wall, the path of sound transmission, and the sound's location.

3. Normal breath sounds are produced by air flow patterns, by associated pressure changes within the airways, and by solid tissue vibrations.

4. Tracheal and mainstem bronchi breath sounds are heard over the chest wall on either side of the sternum from the second intercostal space to the fourth intercostal space anteriorly and along the vertebral column from the third intercostal space to the sixth intercostal space posteriorly. These sounds have a variable pitch and a loud intensity heard best with the diaphragm of the stethoscope. They are heard throughout inspiration and expiration.

5. These normal breath sounds are heard throughout the chest anteriorly, posteriorly, and laterally. Their duration varies, depending on their location, but inspiration is usually followed immediately by a shorter expiration. The sounds have a low pitch that can be heard with either the diaphragm or bell of the stethoscope.

6. Variations in intensity are most often related to airflow patterns and to the distribution of ventilation throughout the lungs. During inspiration, with the patient in the upright position, air flows initially into the lung apices, then into the lung bases (the de-

pendent areas) after the small airways reopen; therefore, intensity will probably be greater in the apices
than in the bases. During normal breathing, this
change in intensity may not always be audible.

7. Intensity may increase during systole because ventricular contraction allows the surrounding lung tissue to expand more fully, increasing turbulent airflow
to that region and intensifying the inspiratory sounds.
Conversely, intensity may decrease during diastole
because ventricular expansion of the heart compresses
adjacent lung tissue, reducing airflow to that region.

8. Normal breath sounds heard at the mouth are thought
to be produced by turbulent airflow occurring below
the glottis and before the terminal airways. In healthy
individuals, breath sounds at the mouth provide baseline data that can be useful later when evaluating
noisy or paradoxically quiet breath sounds.

4 Bronchial breath sounds

1. When lung tissue between the central airways and
the chest wall becomes airless because of conditions
that increase lung density, transmission of breath
sounds from large airways is enhanced.

2. Breath sounds are enhanced over an area of increased
lung density because very little high-frequency sound
is lost through attenuation or filtration. As the lung
tissue density increases the impedance between the
fluid-filled lung tissue and the pleurae and chest wall,
these three media become well matched. This match
decreases the normal filtering of high-frequency
sounds. Consequently, the breath sounds are transmitted more readily to the chest wall surface and are
louder and more tubular than normal breath sounds
heard over the same chest wall area.

3. Conditions associated with bronchial breath sounds
include consolidation, atelectasis, and fibrosis.

4. Clinical findings will vary, depending on the location
of the consolidated area and the causative agent. But
when classic consolidation is present, decreased chest
wall movement and a dull percussion note will be apparent over the affected area.

5. Bronchial breathing will be heard over a dense, airless upper lobe even without a patent bronchus, because the upper lobe surfaces are in direct contact
with the trachea and loud tracheal breath sounds are

transmitted directly to the dense, airless upper lobe tissues. In contrast, bronchial breath sounds will be heard over a dense, airless lower lobe only when the bronchi are patent, because sound is not transmitted directly to the airless lower lobe tissues.

6. Bronchial breath sounds heard over a consolidated area are high-pitched and have the typical hollow, or tubular, quality of normal central airway breath sounds. They remain audible during both expiration and inspiration, but the expiratory sounds are longer and louder when the patient is sitting up. The I:E ratio is 1:2. These sounds may be auscultated with either the bell or diaphragm of the stethoscope.

7. Atelectasis, incomplete expansion of a lung area, is thought to result from uncleared secretions that become thick, occluding the airway.

8. Bronchial breath sounds heard over an atelectatic area are high-pitched and have the typical hollow, or tubular, quality of normal central airway breath sounds. They are audible throughout inspiration and expiration. When the patient is in the supine position, the inspiratory and expiratory sounds are equal in duration and intensity. The I:E ratio is 1:1. These sounds can be heard equally well with either the bell or diaphragm of the stethoscope.

9. Bronchial breath sounds heard over a fibrotic area have the typical hollow, or tubular, quality of normal central airway breath sounds. They are audible throughout inspiration and expiration. When the patient is in the upright position, the breath sounds become progressively louder during inspiration and become both louder and longer during expiration. The I:E ratio is 1:1 to 1:2. These bronchial breath sounds are high-pitched and are heard equally well with either the diaphragm or bell of the stethoscope.

5 Abnormal voice sounds

1. Voice sounds are produced by vibrations of the vocal cords as air from the lungs passes over them. The resonance of the mouth, nasopharynx, and paranasal sinuses helps to amplify these sounds.

2. Transmitted voice sounds are normally heard as a low-pitched, unintelligible mumble over healthy lung and pleural surfaces because most of the vowels are filtered out.

3. Voice sounds are heard distinctly over consolidated or atelectatic lung tissue areas because less filtering takes place, enhancing transmission.
4. Bronchophony is the clear, distinct, intelligible voice sound heard over dense, airless lung tissue. Dense, airless lung tissue transmits high-frequency vowel sounds more easily because of impedance matching. Also, consolidation increases vocal resonance, which allows the clear transmission of voice sounds to the chest wall.
5. Bronchophony is heard over dense, airless upper lobes because the upper lobe surfaces are in direct contact with the trachea, leading to direct transmission of tracheal breath sounds. In contrast, bronchophony is heard over dense, airless lower lobes only when the bronchi are patent because a direct path of sound transmission to the lower lobes doesn't exist.
6. Bronchophony can be heard anywhere over the anterior, lateral, and posterior chest wall surfaces. It is commonly heard over dense, airless lung tissue in the upper lobes, such as a consolidated area.
7. The patient is asked to repeat the words "ninety-nine" several times. Over healthy lung tissue, the words are unintelligible; however, over a consolidated area, the high-frequency sounds are easily understood as words.
8. Whispered pectoriloquy is the clear, distinct, intelligible whispered voice sound heard over airless, consolidated, or atelectatic lung tissue. In a healthy person, normal lung tissue filters the high frequencies of whispered vowel sounds, making them unintelligible during auscultation. But in a patient with consolidation or atelectasis, these same whispered vowel sounds are transmitted to the chest wall surface without much filtering of high frequencies and can be heard clearly with the stethoscope.
9. Whispered pectoriloquy can be heard anywhere over the anterior or posterior chest wall surfaces over dense, airless lung tissue, typically over an area of consolidation or atelectasis.
10. The patient is asked to whisper the words "one-two-three" several times. Over healthy lung tissue, the words are unintelligible; over the atelectatic area, the high-frequency vowel sounds are easily understood as words.
11. Egophony, a voice sound that has a nasal or bleating quality when heard over the chest wall, is produced

over consolidated and atelectatic areas because impedance matching enhances breath sound transmission in such areas. It's also detectable over the upper border of large pleural effusions.

12. Egophony can be heard anywhere over the anterior, posterior, or lateral chest wall surfaces over a consolidated or atelectatic area.

13. The patient is asked to repeat the letter "E" several times. Over healthy lung tissue, the letter sounds as it normally does; over the consolidated area, it sounds like "A-aay" and has a high-pitched, nasal quality.

14. Bronchial breath sounds, bronchophony, whispered pectoriloquy, and egophony are typical in patients with consolidation.

6 Absent and diminished breath sounds

1. Breath sounds are diminished or eliminated by conditions that limit airflow into lung segments. Slow inspiratory airflow rates decrease breath sound amplitude because less air movement occurs, resulting in less turbulent airflow. Diminished or absent breath sounds can also occur when breath sounds are reflected at the visceral and parietal pleurae because of an impedance mismatch.

2. Conditions associated with absent or diminished breath sounds include shallow breathing, diaphragmatic paralysis, severe airway obstruction, pneumothorax, pleural effusion, hyperinflated lungs, and obesity. The use of positive end-expiratory pressure during assisted ventilation is also associated with diminished breath sounds.

3. During normal breathing in the upright position, a certain amount of air flows through the airways during inspiration and expiration; the distribution of ventilation is greater in dependent lung regions because more respiratory movement occurs. During shallow breathing, less respiratory movement occurs; consequently, less air flows through the airways during inspiration and expiration. Because of this reduced airflow, turbulence is decreased and breath sounds are diminished.

4. When the diaphragm becomes paralyzed, as in a patient with a mediastinal tumor, it no longer participates in normal breathing. The internal and external intercostal muscles, which also have a role in normal

breathing, must take over the work of breathing. With only the chest wall muscles initiating the respiratory cycle, ventilation of the lung bases may be limited, resulting in diminished breath sounds.

5. If a lobar or segmental bronchus becomes obstructed, as in a patient who has aspirated a foreign object, airflow ceases distal to the obstruction; therefore, breath sounds will be absent over the area distal to the obstruction. If a mainstem bronchus is obstructed, breath sounds will be absent throughout the affected lung.

6. Breath sounds heard over a pneumothorax are significantly diminished or absent because of acoustical mismatching of the air-filled lung and the collection of air in the pleural space.

7. Diminished or absent breath sounds resulting from a pneumothorax can be heard anywhere over the anterior, posterior, and lateral chest wall surfaces, depending on the location and size of the pneumothorax. Normal breath sounds are heard on the contralateral side over healthy lung tissue, and breath sounds are absent over the pneumothorax. If diminished breath sounds are heard, they have a low pitch that is heard with either the bell or diaphragm of the stethoscope.

8. In pleural effusion, fluid accumulates in the pleural space, impairing the transmission of normal breath sounds.

9. A large pleural effusion compresses adjacent lung tissue, causing atelectasis. The percussion tone will be dull. Egophony, bronchophony, and whispered pectoriloquy caused by the atelectasis may be audible at the upper border of the pleural effusion. Occasionally, very loud bronchial breath sounds may have sufficient intensity to be transmitted through a small pleural effusion.

10. Diminished or absent breath sounds resulting from a pleural effusion may be heard anywhere over the anterior, posterior, or lateral chest wall surfaces, depending on the location of the pleural effusion. Normal breath sounds are heard on the contralateral side over healthy lung tissue. The diminished breath sounds have a low pitch that can be heard with either the bell or diaphragm of the stethoscope.

11. Premature dynamic compression of the large central airways and the loss of elastic tension in the lung tissue limit airflow during expiration. Increased intrin-

sic airway resistance may also be present. Increased amounts of air trapped in the lungs change the acoustical qualities of the sound transmitted, creating a mismatch between the pleurae and chest wall and the hyperinflated lung tissue. Consequently, breath sounds are diminished.

12. Diminished or absent breath sounds associated with chronic obstructive pulmonary disease are heard over the anterior, posterior, and lateral chest wall surfaces. If the breath sounds are audible, they are soft in intensity and have a low pitch heard best with the diaphragm of the stethoscope. The sounds are heard throughout inspiration and expiration.

13. Breath sounds are normally attenuated and filtered at the pleural surface. In an obese person, a thickened chest wall increases the distance between lung tissue and the chest wall surface. This results in additional filtering of the breath sounds as they are transmitted from the pleurae to the chest wall surface.

14. Adding positive end-expiratory pressure (PEEP) during mechanical ventilation of an intubated patient can diminish breath sounds in the following way: PEEP increases functional residual capacity (FRC), the amount of air remaining in the airways at the end of normal expiration. Increasing FRC hyperinflates the lungs. Increased amounts of air in the small airways and alveoli change the acoustical qualities of the sound transmitted through the chest wall, creating a mismatch between the pleurae and chest wall and the hyperinflated lung.

7 Classifying adventitious sounds

1. In 1977, the American Thoracic Society adopted a system of classifying adventitious sounds based on acoustical qualities, timing, and frequency waveforms.

2. Adventitious sounds are classified as crackles and wheezes.

3. Coarse crackles are discontinuous, explosive sounds that are loud and low-pitched.

4. Fine crackles are discontinuous, explosive sounds that are shorter in duration, higher in pitch, and less intense than coarse crackles.

5. Wheezes are continuous sounds that are high-pitched and have a hissing or coughing sound. They often have a musical quality.

6. Low-pitched wheezes are continuous sounds that are low-pitched and often resemble snoring.

8 Adventitious sounds: Crackles

1. Crackles are short, explosive or popping sounds that are described according to their pitch, timing, and location.
2. Two different mechanisms are thought to generate crackles: air bubbling through secretions and the sudden explosive opening of airways.
3. Air bubbling through secretions in the airways is widely accepted as one way crackles are produced. According to Forgacs, this explanation is probably true when the trachea and mainstem bronchi are full of sputum, as commonly occurs with severe pulmonary edema and chronic bronchitis.
4. The sudden opening of multiple collapsed peripheral airways and the associated explosive changes in air pressures are thought to produce the crackles heard over the lung bases in a healthy person who inhales deeply after a maximum exhalation.
5. The timing of crackles is described as early, mid-, or late inspiration or expiration. Pitch is usually described as high or low. Intensity is variable and is described as loud or soft. Density is described as profuse or scanty. Duration, indicating the length of time that the crackles can be heard during inspiration or expiration, varies.
6. Conditions associated with late inspiratory crackles include atelectasis, resolving lobar pneumonia, interstitial fibrosis, and left ventricular failure.
7. Crackles associated with atelectasis are produced by the sudden opening of collapsed small airways and adjoining alveoli.
8. The crackles associated with atelectasis begin late in inspiration and become more profuse toward the end of inspiration. They vary in intensity but are high-pitched. Because crackles associated with atelectasis are poorly transmitted to the chest wall surface, their intensity and density change when the stethoscope is moved only a short distance. They are not audible at the mouth. The patient's position also affects these crackles. For example, in an immobile patient, profuse crackles are heard in the dependent lung regions, but crackles are absent or scanty in non-

dependent lung regions. Also, crackles associated with atelectasis may clear somewhat with coughing.

9. In patients with resolving lobar pneumonia, crackles can be auscultated over lung areas where many alveoli are still filled with exudate, but the surrounding alveoli are aerated and have higher-than-normal ventilation. A large increase in air pressure gradients in the airways reaching these unaerated alveoli generates crackles as the airways are snapped open during late inspiration.

10. Crackles associated with lobar pneumonia begin late in inspiration and become more profuse toward the end of inspiration. These crackles are typically high-pitched.

11. Diffuse interstitial fibrosis impairs or destroys alveoli by filling them with abnormal cells or by scarring the lung tissue. Unaffected alveoli are usually hyperaerated. The lungs become stiff and more difficult to inflate, and airflow volumes usually decrease. Theoretically, the delayed opening of small airways during inspiration causes alveolar pressures in the affected lung tissue to fall more significantly than in healthy alveoli. This fall in alveolar pressures leads to an increased pressure gradient that generates repetitive late inspiratory crackles.

12. As interstitial fibrosis worsens, crackles are heard bilaterally over the posterior lung bases and spread upward toward the apices. In later stages of the disease, crackles aren't affected by position changes and may be heard throughout inspiration.

13. Crackles associated with interstitial fibrosis have a fine intensity and a short, discontinuous duration; they are heard during late inspiration. They have a high pitch heard best with the diaphragm of the stethoscope.

14. Left-sided heart failure leads to fluid accumulation in the lung interstitium.

   Crackles are produced by the rapid equalization of pressures associated with the delayed opening of airways narrowed by pulmonary edema.

15. Crackles associated with early left-sided failure and pulmonary edema are heard bilaterally over the posterior lung bases. However, as pulmonary edema worsens, the crackles become more profuse and may be heard throughout the chest during late inspiration. Their intensity is fine in the early stages of left-sided failure but changes to a loud rattling sound as the patient's condition worsens. Their duration varies with the degree of left-sided failure. They have a low pitch

that's heard best with either the bell or diaphragm of the stethoscope.

16. Coarse crackles are thought to be produced by the intermittent closure of large bronchi and the corresponding flow of a bolus of air through the obstructed area.

17. Early inspiratory crackles are associated with excessive mucus production in patients with chronic bronchitis. The proliferation and hypertrophy of mucous glands within the airways arc caused by chronic exposure to airway irritants, such as cigarette smoke and air pollution.

18. In patients with chronic bronchitis. crackles are heard early in inspiration over all chest wall surfaces and at the mouth. They are scanty and low-pitched and are not affected by the patient's position.

19. Bronchiectasis, irreversible dilatation of the bronchi in selected lung segments, is characterized by chronic and copious production of yellow or green sputum and by fibrotic or atelectatic lung tissue surrounding the affected airways.

20. In patients with bronchiectasis, crackles tend to be profuse, low-pitched, heard during early or midinspiration, and coarser than those associated with chronic bronchitis. Coughing may decrease the number of crackles heard, but position changes do not affect them.

21. When the visceral and parietal pleural surfaces are damaged by fibrin deposits or inflammatory or neoplastic cells, they lose their ability to glide silently over each other during breathing, and their movements become jerky and periodically delayed. This motion produces loud, grating crackles known as pleural crackles or pleural friction rub.

22. Pleural crackles are heard on the chest wall over the affected area. Their intensity is loud, and they have a coarse, grating quality and a low pitch. Their duration is discontinuous. They may be heard during inspiration only or during both the inspiratory and expiratory phases of the respiratory cycle.

9 Adventitious sounds: Wheezes

1. Wheezes are musical sounds generated by air passing through a bronchus so narrowed as to be almost closed. The bronchus walls oscillate between closed and barely open positions; these oscillations generate audible sounds.

2. Wheezes are high-pitched, continuous sounds with frequencies of 200 Hz or greater and a duration of 250 msec or more. Their duration is long enough to carry an audible pitch similar to a musical tone. Wheezes are described by their timing within the respiratory cycle: They may be heard during inspiration, expiration, or continuously throughout the respiratory cycle. They can be further described as localized or diffuse, episodic or chronic.

3. The pitch is determined by the emitted sound's frequency, which can vary widely over a five-octave range. These differences in frequency are attributed to the airway size and elasticity and to airflow rates through the narrowed bronchus.

4. Wheezes are transmitted better through airways than through lung tissue, which absorbs high-frequency sounds.

5. Conditions associated with wheezes include bronchospasm, airway thickening caused by mucosal swelling or muscle hypertrophy, inhalation of a foreign object, tumor, secretions, or dynamic airway compression.

6. Polyphonic wheezes are believed to be caused by the dynamic compression of large airways during expiration. In healthy individuals, polyphonic wheezes can sometimes be auscultated during a maximal forced expiration when the dynamic compression occurs simultaneously in all airways.

7. In patients with widespread air-flow obstruction, elastic recoil properties, peripheral airway resistance, and airway mechanics are altered throughout both lungs. Together these abnormal changes affect the timing of dynamic airway compression within the bronchi. This change in airway compression alters normal sound production.

8. Expiratory polyphonic wheezes are usually heard over the anterior, posterior, and lateral chest wall surfaces during expiration. Their intensity is usually described as loud and musical, and their duration is continuous. They have a high pitch heard best with the diaphragm of the stethoscope.

9. Fixed monophonic wheezes, which have a constant pitch and a single musical tone, are generated by the oscillations of a large, partially obstructed bronchus. The obstruction may be caused by a tumor, a foreign body, bronchial stenosis, or an intrabronchial granuloma.

10. Fixed monophonic wheezes are heard over the anterior, posterior, and right lateral chest wall surfaces. These wheezes are usually loud, and their duration is continuous. They may be heard during inspiration, expiration, or throughout the respiratory cycle. They have a low pitch heard best with the diaphragm of the stethoscope.

11. Sequential inspiratory wheezes are sometimes heard over the lung bases in patients with interstitial fibrosis, asbestosis, or fibrosing alveolitis.

12. These monophonic wheezes are generated by airways that open late in inspiration in unaerated lung regions. The rapid inflow of air precipitates airway wall vibrations, generating sequential inspiratory wheezes.

13. Sequential inspiratory wheezes are usually heard over the lateral and posterior lung bases. They have a loud intensity and a continuous duration. They occur throughout inspiration but are more predominant in late inspiration. They have a high pitch heard best with the diaphragm of the stethoscope.

14. Airways narrowed by bronchospasm or mucosal swelling produce single or multiple monophonic wheezes that may occur during inspiration, expiration, or throughout the respiratory cycle.

15. Random monophonic wheezes are typically heard in patients with severe status asthmaticus.

16. The progressive airway obstruction that occurs in patients with status asthmaticus can cause a dynamic pattern of wheezing. First, monophonic wheezes are heard only during expiration; then they are heard throughout the respiratory cycle. As status asthmaticus becomes more severe, all wheezes heard over the chest wall surfaces disappear because a combination of air trapping and severe airway narrowing causes the site of dynamic airway compression to move toward the lung periphery. This phenomenon is called a silent chest.

17. Random monophonic wheezes are usually heard over the anterior, posterior, and lateral chest wall surfaces. They are usually loud, and their duration is continuous. These wheezes occur throughout the respiratory cycle, and expiration is frequently prolonged. They have a high pitch heard best with the diaphragm of the stethoscope.

18. Stridor is a very loud musical sound that is heard at a distance from the patient, usually without a stethoscope.

19. Stridor is caused by laryngeal spasm and mucosal swelling, which contract the vocal cords and narrow the airway.
20. Severe stridor is heard without a stethoscope; however, in a patient with a less pronounced laryngeal spasm, stridor may be heard by auscultating over the larynx. Stridor is very loud and has a continuous duration. It may be heard during inspiration or throughout the respiratory cycle. Its high pitch resembles a crowing sound.

Heart sounds

10 The heart and auscultation

1. The heart's primary function is to pump deoxygenated blood to the lungs, where carbon dioxide–oxygen (CO_2-O_2) exchange takes place, and to pump oxygenated blood throughout the body.
2. The top, or superior, part of the heart is called the base; the most inferior and lateral part of the heart is called the apex.
3. Anatomically, the heart is divided into two functional sides: the right side and the left side, which are separated by the septum. Each side is further divided into chambers. The right atrium and right ventricle are the right-sided chambers; the left atrium and left ventricle are the left-sided chambers.
4. The right atrioventricular, or tricuspid, valve separates the right atrium and right ventricle, and the left atrioventricular, or mitral, valve separates the left atrium and left ventricle. The semilunar pulmonic valve separates the right ventricle and pulmonary artery, and the semilunar aortic valve separates the left ventricle and aorta.
5. Deoxygenated, or venous, blood from nearly every tissue of the body flows into the right atrium via the superior and inferior venae cavae. Venous blood from the heart tissues itself drains via the coronary sinus directly into the right atrium. The deoxygenated blood collects there until the tricuspid valve opens. Then the deoxygenated blood flows into the right ventricle. From the right ventricle, it flows through the open pulmonic valve into the pulmonary artery, which distributes deoxygenated blood to both lungs.

The complex process of carbon dioxide–oxygen exchange occurs in the alveoli. Then the oxygenated blood flows back to the heart via the pulmonary veins and collects in the left atrium. From there, oxygenated blood flows through the opened mitral valve into the left ventricle. When the aortic valve opens, oxygenated blood flows into the aorta, which transports it to all body tissues.

6. A healthy heart in a 154-lb (70-kg) adult pumps approximately 1⅝ gal (6 L) of blood per minute. Because the total blood volume in a healthy adult is about 1⅜ gal (5.2 L), the heart pumps the body's total blood volume in less than 1 minute.

7. During systole, heart muscle contraction raises the intracardiac pressures enough to systematically open the valves and pump a certain volume of blood. During diastole, the heart muscle relaxes, allowing the chambers to fill with blood again. This entire sequence is called the cardiac cycle.

8. Cardiac output is the amount of blood pumped into the aorta each minute; it's highly dependent on stroke volume. Stroke volume is the amount of blood pumped during each ventricular contraction.

9. Electrical impulses are primarily responsible for the heart's rhythmic pumping action. These impulses are discharged automatically from specialized cardiac cells that stimulate the heart muscle to contract. The specialized cardiac cells and fibers within the conduction system work together to produce a contraction. The impulses fired from the sinoatrial (SA) node, located just below the entrance of the superior vena cava in the right atrium, normally initiate the cardiac cycle, and they usually travel along specific pathways. For example, when the electrical impulse leaves the SA node, it travels along the atrial conduction pathways located in the atrial walls, initiating atrial systole (or atrial contraction). The impulse very rapidly reaches the atrioventricular (AV) node, located near the AV junction. From the AV node, the impulse travels to the bundle of His located in the interventricular septum. Here the bundle of His divides into the right and left bundle branches. These branches further divide into the tiny Purkinje fibers located throughout the ventricular walls. As the impulse travels through the bundle branches and Purkinje fibers, it initiates ventricular systole (or ventricular contraction).

10. The sequential and synchronized contraction (systole) and relaxation (diastole) of the atria and ventricles, along with the opening and closing of competent, properly functioning valves, ensure a unidirectional flow of blood through the heart and allow the heart to effectively move blood to all areas of the body quickly and repeatedly.

11. The aortic area is located at the second right intercostal space close to the sternal border. Abbreviated as 2RSB, this area is where sounds of the aortic valve and aorta are heard best.

   The pulmonic area is located at the second left intercostal space close to the sternal border. Abbreviated as 2LSB, this area is where the pulmonic valve and pulmonary artery sounds are heard best.

   The tricuspid area is located at the fifth left intercostal space close to the sternal border. This area, abbreviated as 5LSB, is where sounds of the tricuspid valve and right ventricle are heard best.

   The mitral area is located at or near the fifth intercostal space just medial to the left midclavicular line. This area, directly over the left ventricle, is sometimes referred to as the apical area, or apex. The mitral area, abbreviated as 5LMCL, is where sounds associated with the mitral valve and left ventricle are heard best.

   Erb's point differs from the four other areas in that it is not named after a heart valve, but it is a good location to hear sounds of aortic and pulmonic origin. Abbreviated as 3LSB, this area is located at the third left intercostal space close to the sternal border.

12. The chest piece should have a diaphragm and a bell. The diaphragm is designed to transmit high-pitched sounds more clearly, and the bell is designed to transmit low-pitched sounds more clearly. A flat, adult-sized diaphragm should be approximately 1⅜″ (3.5 cm) in diameter and should be smooth, thin, and stiff enough to filter out low-frequency sounds. The bell should be approximately 1″ (2.5 cm) in diameter and deep enough so that it does not fill with tissue when placed on the chest wall. The tubing length can vary from 10″ to 15″ (25 to 38 cm), and its inside diameter should be ⅛″ — or ³⁄₁₆″ if the tubing is longer. The earpieces should fit inside the ears comfortably, and the stethoscope should not be too heavy because its weight can interfere with your ability to hear sounds accurately.

13. To use the diaphragm, firmly grasp the metal area between the bell and the diaphragm with your finger and thumb, and press down firmly on the chest wall. Or place your fingertips on the bell's rim, and press down firmly against the chest wall. Apply enough pressure so that an indentation remains on the skin after you remove the stethoscope.

    The bell, however, should touch the chest wall only lightly. If you exert too much pressure when listening with the bell, the stretched skin beneath it will act as a diaphragm, filtering out low-pitched sounds. To hold the bell correctly, grasp the diaphragm's outer edges with the index finger and thumb, and gently rest the bell on the chest wall. Look at the skin around the edges of the bell to see if too much pressure is being applied. If any signs of indentation appear on the skin, relax the downward pressure.

14. Listen first with the diaphragm over the aortic area. Try to recognize the characteristic lub-dub sound of each cardiac cycle. After listening through several cycles, inch the diaphragm toward the pulmonic area. Try to move the diaphragm without losing track of the lub-dub. Then listen over the pulmonic area, Erb's point, and the tricuspid area. Continue in this manner until you reach the mitral area.

15. To locate the point of maximum impulse (PMI), turn the patient slightly to the left, placing him in the partial left lateral recumbent position. This position brings the heart's apex closer to the chest wall. Closely observe the chest wall for any sign of the heartbeat, which may appear as a rhythmic bulging. Then use your fingertip pads to palpate for the heartbeat between the fourth and sixth intercostal spaces, near the left midclavicular line. The chest wall site where the heartbeat is seen and felt is the PMI.

16. Several maneuvers can enhance the heart sounds heard during auscultation. For example, you can have the patient squat or stand, hold his breath, or raise his legs while in a supine position. Another common technique is to have the patient cough several times or perform Valsalva's maneuver. During this maneuver, the patient attempts to exhale forcefully against a closed glottis.

    Another method that enhances the sounds heard during auscultation is to have the patient increase the depth of breathing. This decreases the respiratory rate and makes it easier to distinguish sounds originating in either the right or left side of the heart. For example, during inspiration, venous return is enhanced, accentuating right-sided cardiac events; during expiration, left-sided blood flow is enhanced, accentuating left-sided cardiac events.

You can help the patient by raising your hand slowly when you want him to inhale, then lowering your hand slowly when you want him to exhale. Caution the patient to breathe smoothly and continuously. Breath holding may produce a Valsalva-type maneuver, which will negate the cardiac responses being assessed.

11 Heart sound dynamics

1. The heart sounds heard through a stethoscope during auscultation are generated by vibrations from the heart's walls and valves and from turbulent blood flow.
2. At the beginning of ventricular diastole, the ventricles are relaxed, and the aortic valve closes slightly before the pulmonic valve. For a brief time, both the atrioventricular and semilunar valves are closed. During this period, called isovolumic relaxation, intraventricular pressures continue to fall. But the opening of the tricuspid and mitral valves follows quickly, and blood begins to flow passively from the atria into the ventricles. As the ventricles become distended, the rate of ventricular filling decreases.
3. When the atria contract (from stimulation of the atrial myocardium by an electrical impulse from the sinoatrial node), a slight boost in ventricular volume occurs. The resulting increase in ventricular pressures causes the mitral and tricuspid valves to begin closing. During atrial systole, the electrical impulse moves more slowly through the atrioventricular node and into the bundle of His. The impulse proceeds rapidly through the bundle branches and the Purkinje fibers, activating ventricular systole.
4. Early in ventricular systole, intraventricular pressures increase above intra-atrial pressures, and the mitral and tricuspid valves close suddenly. Normally, the mitral valve closes slightly before the tricuspid valve. For another brief period, both the atrioventricular and semilunar valves are closed. During this period, known as isovolumic contraction, ventricular pres-

sures increase, becoming higher than the pressures in the pulmonary artery and aorta. The aortic and pulmonic valves open, and blood is ejected through them. Normally, the aortic valve opens slightly before the pulmonic valve.

After a period of maximum ejection of blood from the ventricles, the ventricles begin to relax. As intraventricular pressures fall rapidly, a brief backflow of blood from the pulmonary artery and aorta toward the ventricles occurs. Reduced intraventricular pressures and the temporary backflow of blood are associated with closure of the aortic and pulmonic valves at the end of systole.

5. S_1, the first heart sound, is heard at the beginning of systole. It's associated with closure of the mitral and tricuspid valves and the increasing pressures within the ventricles that cause the moving valve leaflets and cord structures to decelerate. S_1 is generated by the closing atrioventricular valves and the vibrations caused by tensing of the chordae tendineae.

6. At the end of ventricular systole, ventricular pressures fall rapidly, causing a slight backflow of blood from the aorta and pulmonary artery. The decrease in ventricular pressures to a level below that of aortic and pulmonic systolic pressures and the temporary backflow of blood and recoil events are associated with closure of the aortic and pulmonic valves. The vibrations associated with these events produce the second heart sound, S_2, which marks the end of ventricular systole.

7. A sound's location is the anatomic area on the patient's chest wall where the sound is heard best. Bony structures and landmarks, such as the right and left midclavicular lines, are used to describe the precise location.

8. Intensity refers to the sound's loudness during auscultation. Usually, a sound's intensity is determined somewhat subjectively, based on experience. However, when abnormalities are present, intensity can be determined electronically by recording a phonocardiogram and measuring the amplitude of the sound's vibrations.

9. Sound duration refers to the length of time the sound is heard; it can be described as either short or long. A sound's duration affects whether you hear it as a click, a snap, or a murmur.

10. A sound's pitch is determined by the frequency of its vibrations. High-frequency sounds, like the notes of a piccolo, are best heard with the diaphragm of the stethoscope; low-frequency sounds, like the notes of a tuba, are best heard with the bell of the stethoscope.

11. Sound quality is determined by the combination of its frequencies. It may be described as sharp, dull, booming, snapping, blowing, harsh, or musical.

12. A sound's timing refers to when it is heard during the cardiac cycle (during systole or diastole).

13. The sequential and rhythmic process of depolarization and repolarization is referred to as the heart's electrical activity. Electrical activity occurs at the cellular level in every contractile cell of the myocardium. Initially, the contractile cell is polarized (in a resting state). Depolarization begins when the cell membrane becomes permeable to the flow of sodium ions into the cell. Repolarization begins when calcium ions move into the cell and potassium ions begin to move out of the cell. Then the accumulated intracellular sodium and calcium ions are extruded while the lost potassium is restored to the cell by the sodium-potassium pump, completing repolarization. The cell is polarized to its original ionic state, and the myocardium relaxes.

14. The electrocardiogram (ECG) correlates with the heart's electrical activity in the following manner. The sinoatrial node fires, triggering an atrial contraction. The P wave, part of the ECG waveform, represents atrial depolarization. The QRS complex represents electrical depolarization of the ventricles. Atrial repolarization is not seen in the ECG because it is hidden in the PR segment and the QRS complex. The T wave represents ventricular repolarization. The impulse travels through the atrioventricular node, the bundle of His, the bundle branches, and the Purkinje fibers before the ventricles contract. The time between atrial contraction and ventricular contraction is recorded in the ECG as the PR interval: It begins at the onset of the P wave and lasts until the onset of the QRS complex.

15. The first (S_1) and second (S_2) heart sounds directly correlate with a patient's ECG. S_1 normally occurs just after the QRS complex; S_2 occurs at the end of the T wave.

16. The intensity, duration, and timing of heart sounds can be represented graphically as rectangular blocks

placed perpendicularly on a horizontal baseline. The block's height corresponds to the heart sound's intensity (the higher the intensity, the higher the block); the block's width corresponds to the sound's duration. The proximity of one block on the baseline to the next block represents the time interval between one sound and another. The spacing between the blocks can also be used to specify the relationship of a particular heart sound to systole or diastole.

12 The first heart sound

1. The vibrations associated with closure of the mitral and tricuspid valves produce the first heart sound, S_1.

2. Normally, only two components of the first heart sound are audible. The first component, referred to as M_1, is associated with closure of the mitral valve; the second component, T_1, is associated with closure of the tricuspid valve. Both valves close at the beginning of ventricular systole, but the mitral valve usually closes slightly ahead of the tricuspid valve.

3. M_1 and T_1 are usually perceived as a single sound called S_1, which is heard best near the heart's apex over the mitral area using the diaphragm of the stethoscope. A single sound is heard because left heart sounds are normally more intense at this site. S_1 occurs shortly after the beginning of the QRS complex in the ECG wave-form. As you inch the stethoscope from the mitral area toward the tricuspid area, without losing track of S_1, the M_1 and T_1 components of S_1 become evident. Expiration makes them easier to hear. T_1 trails M_1 slightly and is softer; it's heard best near the left sternal border. The timing of M_1 and T_1 with the QRS complex remains the same.

4. S_1 is usually heard best near the heart's apex over the mitral area. Its intensity directly relates to the force of ventricular contraction and the amount of ventricular pressure developed during systole. S_1 is short in duration. You can hear its high pitch best with the diaphragm of the stethoscope. The quality of S_1 is somewhat dull. S_1 timing coincides with the beginning of ventricular systole and just precedes a palpable carotid pulse.

5. S_1 can be enhanced by sympathetic stimulation such as that provided by a brief period of exercise.

6. The normal M_1–T_1 split heard over the tricuspid area widens when electrical activation and contraction of the right ventricle are delayed. Such a delay causes delayed tricuspid valve closure.

7. Conditions associated with an abnormal S_1 split are complete right bundle-branch block, left ventricular ectopic beats, epicardial pacing of the left ventricle, and left ventricular tachycardia.

13 The second heart sound

1. The vibrations associated with closure of the aortic and pulmonic valves produce the second heart sound, S_2.

2. S_2, like S_1, has two basic components: the aortic (A_2) component and the pulmonic (P_2) component. Both of these valves close at the end of ventricular systole. Normally, the aortic valve closes slightly ahead of the pulmonic valve.

3. To hear both components of S_2, listen carefully with the diaphragm of the stethoscope over the pulmonic area. Listen for S_2 just after the T wave in the patient's ECG.

4. S_2 is usually heard best near the heart's base over the pulmonic area or over Erb's point. Its intensity directly relates to the amount of closing pressure in the aorta and pulmonary artery. S_2 is slightly shorter in duration than S_1. You can hear its high pitch best with the diaphragm of the stethoscope. The quality of S_2 is somewhat booming; its timing coincides with the end of ventricular systole.

5. The splitting of S_2 into the A_2 and P_2 components is heard best during inspiration over Erb's point. Remember, inspiration causes an increase in venous return to the right side of the heart. This increased venous return prolongs right ventricular ejection time, thus delaying P_2, or closure of the pulmonic valve. A decrease in blood flow to the left side of the heart occurs simultaneously, resulting in a shorter left ventricular ejection time. Therefore, A_2 is heard earlier than P_2. This means that a normal S_2 split is heard during inspiration, and the A_2 and P_2 components fuse during expiration.

6. The intensity of A_2 and P_2 changes proportionally with the difference in pressure gradients across the closed aortic and pulmonic valves. For example, P_2 may be louder than normal in conditions associated

with elevated pulmonary artery diastolic pressure, as occurs in some patients with heart failure, mitral stenosis, Eisenmenger's syndrome, or other congenital heart diseases. When P_2 increases in intensity, it is sometimes heard over the mitral area and along the left sternal border.

A_2 intensity increases when diastolic pressure in the aorta increases. This commonly happens during exercise; during states of excitement such as extreme fear; in hyperkinetic conditions, such as thyrotoxicosis, fever, and pregnancy; and in systemic hypertension. However, if the patient has left ventricular decompensation, ventricular relaxation is slower, and the pressure gradients may not be great enough to produce an accentuated A_2.

Conversely, A_2 intensity may be diminished in conditions that alter the development of diastolic pressure gradients, such as aortic regurgitation and hypotension. A_2 intensity also decreases when ventricular dysfunction is present, such as after an acute myocardial infarction. In this condition, P_2 may become louder if pulmonary artery pressure rises and systemic pressure falls.

7. Abnormal splitting is related to valvular dysfunction, to alterations in blood flow to or from the ventricles, or to both. These changes may cause the normal S_2 split to be absent during both phases of the respiratory cycle. Thus, only a single S_2 is heard over Erb's point. In another case, the split sounds may persist through inspiration and expiration with little or no respiratory variation. The split sounds also may be heard paradoxically on expiration. The A_2–P_2 intervals vary, as does the intensity of A_2 and P_2 during the respiratory cycle. Changes in S_2 splits are usually most noticeable at the beginning of inspiration and expiration.

8. The P_2 component may not be heard during auscultation over Erb's point in the patient with severe pulmonic stenosis. Consequently, S_2 remains a single sound during both inspiration and expiration. A normal S_2 split may also be absent if the A_2 sound masks the P_2 sound or vice versa — for example, when one sound is significantly louder than the other, making splitting inaudible. This phenomenon occurs in patients with pulmonary hypertension. On the other hand, systemic hypertension causes A_2 to be delayed and to fuse with P_2 during inspiration.

9. A persistent S_2 split occurs when A_2 and P_2 don't fuse into one sound during expiration, even though some respiratory variation in the intensity of A_2 and P_2 is heard. This persistent A_2–P_2 splitting during expiration usually results from early aortic valve closure or delayed pulmonic valve closure. Early aortic valve closure is associated with shortened left ventricular systole, which occurs in patients with mitral regurgitation, ventricular septal defects, or cardiac tamponade. Delayed pulmonic valve closure occurs when right ventricular systole is prolonged in patients with chronic pulmonary hypertension. In these patients, the A_2–P_2 split is heard, but the interval between the A_2 and P_2 components is narrowed.

   Another cause of persistent A_2–P_2 splitting throughout expiration is delayed electrical activation of the right ventricle, which will delay P_2. This phenomenon is commonly found in patients with right bundle-branch block, left ventricular epicardial pacing, or left ventricular ectopic beats.

10. A prolonged right ventricular ejection time produces expiratory A_2–P_2 splits that are widened and that persist even when the patient is seated. This occurs in patients with atrial septal defects, acute pulmonary hypertension secondary to massive pulmonary emboli, or pulmonic stenosis. The P_2 component may not be audible at all in patients with severe pulmonic stenosis. A wide, fixed S_2 split is sometimes associated with the pulmonary vascular bed's increased capacitance (ability to receive blood volume and the decreased resistance that accompanies it). This phenomenon occurs in patients with idiopathic dilation of the pulmonary artery or with atrial septal defects. This split does not change with respiration.

11. In a paradoxical, or reversed, S_2 split, P_2 precedes A_2 and the split sounds are heard during expiration instead of inspiration. This phenomenon is almost always caused by delayed aortic valve closure. If A_2 is delayed during expiration, it may follow P_2, causing an S_2 split; if A_2 is delayed during inspiration, A_2 and P_2 fuse because inspiration normally delays P_2. Therefore, S_2 is heard as a single sound during inspiration instead of a normally split sound.

   Delayed A_2 is commonly seen in patients with delayed activation of the left ventricle caused by left bundle-branch block. It is also associated with right

ventricular ectopic beats or right ventricular endocardial pacing. Prolonged left ventricular systole can
also cause a delay in A_2. The same paradoxical $P_2 -$
A_2 split may be heard in patients with left ventricular failure or ischemic heart disease.

Left ventricular pressure overload, which occurs
in patients with systemic hypertension and hypertrophic cardiomyopathy, may also cause paradoxical
S_2 split. Likewise, aortic stenosis may lead to paradoxical splitting of A_2 and P_2; however, if the stenosis is severe, the A_2 component may not be audible.
With left ventricular volume overload, which is frequently associated with aortic regurgitation or patent
ductus arteriosus, A_2 may be delayed and a paradoxical S_2 split may be heard.

14 The third and fourth heart sounds

1. The two left ventricular diastolic filling sounds, S_3
   and S_4, are sometimes heard over the mitral area.
   These sounds differ from S_1 and S_2 in that they are
   low-frequency sounds and are produced by ventricular filling rather than by valve closure.
2. Early in diastole, after isovolumic relaxation, the mitral and tricuspid valves open and the ventricles fill
   and expand. In children and young adults, the left ventricle is normally compliant, permitting rapid filling.
   The left ventricle responds to this rapid filling with an
   abrupt change in wall motion that causes a sudden decrease in blood flow. These events generate vibrations
   that are responsible for the physiologic S_3.
3. A physiologic S_3 is commonly audible in patients with
   high-output conditions, in which rapid ventricular
   expansion, caused by increased blood volume, is present. Anemia, fever, pregnancy, and thyrotoxicosis are
   some of the conditions that cause rapid ventricular
   expansion, resulting in an S_3. An S_3 is also commonly
   heard in young, slender individuals during periods of
   excessive catecholamine release.
4. S_3 is usually heard best with the bell of the stethoscope over the mitral area, and it can often be palpated over the same area. It's heard best during expiration, when blood flow into the left ventricle is increased.
5. S_3 is usually heard best near the heart's apex over the
   mitral area. In some patients, it's faint in intensity

and difficult to hear; in others, it may be loud and easy to hear. S_3 has a short duration, and it may occur only intermittently during every third or fourth heartbeat. It has a low pitch that is heard best with the bell of the stethoscope. S_3 usually has a dull, thudlike quality. Its timing is closely related to S_2, which is heard just after the T wave; S_3 follows S_2 by less than 0.20 second.

6. Because S_3 is associated with blood volume and velocity, it can be intensified by maneuvers that increase stroke volume, such as elevating the patient's legs from a recumbent position or having the patient exercise briefly or cough several times. Placing the patient in the partial left lateral recumbent position often enhances your ability to auscultate and palpate an S_3.

7. The differences between the two sounds are related to the patient's age, clinical condition, or both. Also, an S_3 gallop rhythm usually persists despite maneuvers that decrease venous return.

8. An abnormal S_3 is almost always associated with increased mean left atrial pressure caused by a non-compliant left ventricle. This auscultatory finding is heard in patients with hypertrophic cardiomyopathy and frequently indicates elevated left ventricular diastolic pressure, as occurs in patients with heart failure.

An abnormal S_3 may also be heard in conditions associated with increased blood volume and increased inflow velocity into the left ventricle. It's heard with or without an increase in ventricular diastolic pressure. Consequently, patients with mitral regurgitation and constrictive pericarditis will have an abnormal S_3. This heart sound can also be heard during increased blood flow through the mitral valve, which occurs in patients with ventricular septal defects, patent ductus arteriosus, or severe aortic regurgitation.

An abnormal S_3 in patients with constrictive pericarditis is called a pericardial knock. This type of abnormal S_3 occurs closer to S_2. The interval between S_2 and S_3 is usually less than 0.14 second.

9. An S_3 sometimes originates in the right ventricle instead of the left; when it does, it is always considered abnormal. A right-sided S_3 is heard best over the third, fourth, and fifth intercostal spaces along the left sternal border or over the epigastric area. It is more promi-

nent during inspiration because of increased blood flow into the right ventricle.

10. By the end of diastole, the ventricles are nearly full; atrial contraction further stretches and fills the ventricles. The vibrations caused by this filling and stretching in late diastole generate an additional heart sound, S_4, sometimes called an atrial diastolic gallop.

11. S_4 is usually heard best near the heart's apex over the mitral area; occasionally, it's also palpable over this area. In some patients, it's faint in intensity and difficult to hear, but in others it's loud and easily heard. S_4 is relatively short in duration and may occur only intermittently, during every third or fourth heartbeat. It has a low pitch heard best with the bell of the stethoscope and a thudlike quality. Its timing is presystolic: S_4 precedes S_1 and occurs during the PR interval.

12. To enhance S_4, place the patient in the partial left lateral recumbent position, which brings the heart closer to the chest wall.

13. An abnormal S_4 is heard in numerous conditions, including hypertension (the most common cause), hypertrophic cardiomyopathy, and during or after an acute myocardial infarction. When an S_4 is heard in a patient with hypertension, the systolic blood pressure usually exceeds 160 mm Hg or the diastolic pressure exceeds 100 mm Hg. An abnormal S_4 can also accompany volume overload conditions, such as hyperthyroidism, severe anemia, and sudden severe mitral regurgitation.

14. Normally, S_4 precedes S_1 by an appreciable interval that correlates with the PR interval on the ECG. However, in patients with first-degree AV block, the P wave occurs early in diastole, and S_4 may occur during the early rapid diastolic filling period. Likewise, in tachycardia, S_4 may be superimposed on S_3 during early rapid filling. Should either of these conditions exist, the S_4 fuses with S_3 to become a single diastolic filling sound called a summation gallop, which may be louder than S_4, S_3, or S_1.

15. An S_4 generated in the right ventricle is called a right-sided S_4. It's commonly heard in conditions that increase pressure in the right ventricle by more than 100 mm Hg, such as pulmonic stenosis or pulmonary hypertension. This heart sound is heard best over the third, fourth, and fifth intercostal spaces along the left sternal border and over the epigastric area with

the patient in a supine position; it is more audible during inspiration.

16. Distinguishing an S_1 split $(M_1–T_1)$ from an S_4–S_1 sequence is sometimes difficult; however, here are some ways to help you do so. An S_1 split is heard best between the mitral and tricuspid areas with the diaphragm of the stethoscope, whereas an S_4 is heard best over the mitral area with the bell of the stethoscope and is usually not audible with the diaphragm. Also, an S_4 may be palpable and will disappear when the patient stands. The intensity of S_4 can usually be increased by maneuvers that increase venous return to the heart, such as exercising briefly, squatting, or raising the legs while in a recumbent position.

17. S_3, like S_4, is low-pitched and may be faint or loud and heard only intermittently. Both sounds are heard best over the mitral area, using the bell of the stethoscope, with the patient in a partial left lateral recumbent position. Both sounds are intensified by expiration and can be enhanced by maneuvers that increase stroke volume, such as elevating the legs while in a recumbent position. The absence of S_3 and presence of S_4 indicate a compensated cardiac state. However, if the mean left atrial pressure rises, an abnormal S_3 may become audible. This is associated with a more serious prognosis for the patient.

15 Other diastolic and systolic sounds

1. If the mitral valve leaflets become stenotic or abnormally narrowed while remaining somewhat mobile, they create an opening snap (OS).

2. An OS is usually heard best near the heart's apex over the mitral area or just medial to it. Its intensity varies among patients, and it is usually easy to hear during auscultation. An OS has a short duration. It has a high pitch heard best with the diaphragm of the stethoscope and a sharp, snaplike quality. Its timing is closely related to S_2: An OS occurs early in ventricular diastole, just after the stenotic mitral valve opens.

3. One characteristic of an OS that helps distinguish it from P_2 is its timing: The A_2–P_2 interval is normally shorter than the A_2–OS interval. Also, when the patient stands, the A_2–P_2 interval narrows, whereas the A_2–OS interval widens. Another characteristic is that the A_2–OS interval remains constant through-

out respiration, whereas the A_2–P_2 interval normally widens during inspiration and narrows during expiration. During inspiration, three distinct sounds can usually be heard over the pulmonic area; therefore, the sequence must be A_2, P_2, OS. In contrast, during expiration, the A_2–P_2 interval narrows or fuses, forming one sound. This creates an S_2–OS interval. Finally, P_2 is not usually heard over the mitral area, so if you hear a split S_2 over this area, it is likely to be an S_2 and an OS.

4. One characteristic of an OS that helps distinguish it from an S_3 is its timing: The A_2–S_3 interval is usually longer than the A_2–OS interval. Also, S_3 is a low-frequency sound heard best over the mitral area with the bell of the stethoscope. In contrast, an OS produces a high-frequency sound that is more widely transmitted across the precordium and is heard best with the diaphragm.

   Another characteristic of an OS is that its intensity usually isn't affected by having the patient stand, whereas S_3 intensity can be decreased by standing. If the OS is affected, it is intensified. Another way to differentiate S_3 from an OS is by listening for respiratory changes. An S_3 is usually louder during expiration than during inspiration and is often palpable; an OS doesn't vary in intensity with respiration. Finally, if the murmur typically heard in patients with mitral stenosis is present, you can confirm that the sound is an OS.

5. A systolic ejection sound (ES) is usually a brief, high-frequency sound that is heard best with the diaphragm of the stethoscope. It may be heard near the heart's base over the aortic or pulmonic area; over Erb's point; or near the apex over the mitral area. A systolic ES occurs just after the QRS complex in the ECG waveform.

6. A pulmonic ejection sound (PES) is commonly associated with ventricular ejection and the maximum opening of a stenotic, yet mobile, pulmonic valve. It may also be caused by sudden distention of an already dilated pulmonary artery and by forceful ventricular ejection from pulmonary hypertension.

7. A PES is usually heard best near the heart's base over the pulmonic area. Its intensity is soft but may be equal to or greater than that of S_1. A PES has a short duration. It has a high pitch heard best with the diaphragm of the stethoscope and a sharp, or clicklike,

quality. Its timing is closely related to S_1: It occurs early in ventricular systole, just after the opening of a stenotic pulmonic valve, and is heard just after the QRS complex.

8. Unlike a PES, caused by pulmonic valve stenosis, an aortic ejection sound (AES), caused by aortic valve stenosis, does not vary in intensity with respiration.

9. An AES is heard best near the heart's apex over the mitral area, near the heart's base over the aortic area, or over Erb's point. Its intensity is soft but may be equal to or greater than that of S_1. An AES has a short duration. It has a high pitch that is heard best with the diaphragm of the stethoscope and a sharp, or clicklike, quality. Its timing is closely related to S_1. An AES occurs early in ventricular systole, just after the opening of a stenotic aortic valve, and is heard just after the QRS complex in the ECG waveform.

10. Certain characteristics help to distinguish an AES from other heart sounds. One characteristic is that an AES radiates more than a PES. Another characteristic is that a split S_1 heard over the mitral area is likely to be an M_1 and an AES.

   You can differentiate an AES from an S_4 by remembering that S_4 is heard best with the bell of the stethoscope over the mitral area and is frequently accompanied by a palpable, presystolic apical bulge. Also, an S_4 is intensified by maneuvers that increase venous return to the heart, such as brief exercise, squatting, raising the legs from a recumbent position, coughing, or performing Valsalva's maneuver; an AES is not affected by any of these maneuvers.

11. A midsystolic click (MSC) occurs when the prolapsed mitral valve's leaflets and chordae tendineae tense. The anterior or posterior leaflet or both leaflets can prolapse.

12. An MSC is usually heard best over the tricuspid area and near the heart's apex over the mitral area. Its intensity is equal to or greater than that of S_1. An MSC has a short duration. It has a high pitch that is heard best with the diaphragm of the stethoscope, and its quality is clicklike. The click's timing varies: it can occur in early, mid-, or late systole. An MSC can be heard during the QT interval in the ECG waveform.

13. The timing of an MSC is affected by various maneuvers, such as having the patient stand or perform Valsalva's maneuver. Such maneuvers result in reduced left ventricular filling and cause the MSC to be heard

closer to S_1. The MSC may even merge with S_1 and disappear completely. Increasing left ventricular volume by raising the legs from a recumbent position delays the click. This maneuver may also cause the prolapse not to occur and the MSC to be diminished or inaudible. Sometimes an MSC is accompanied by a late systolic crescendo murmur or the characteristic holosystolic murmur of mitral regurgitation. An MSC may also be caused by some extracardiac conditions such as pleuropericardial adhesions.

16 Murmur fundamentals

1. Several clinically significant conditions — such as blood flowing at a high velocity through a partially obstructed opening, blood flowing from a smaller chamber to a larger one, or a combination of these — can cause turbulent blood flow.
2. The terms used to describe a specific characteristic are determined primarily by the volume and speed of the jet of blood as it moves through the heart.
3. The seven characteristics used to describe murmurs are location, intensity, duration, pitch, quality, timing, and configuration.
4. A murmur's location is the anatomic area on the chest wall where the murmur is heard best and is usually also the murmur's point of maximum intensity. This area usually correlates with the underlying location of the valve that is responsible for producing the murmur.
5. The murmur's sounds may also be transmitted to the chamber or vessel where the turbulent blood flow occurs. This phenomenon, known as radiation, occurs because the direction of blood flow determines sound transmission. Murmurs radiate in either a forward or backward direction.
6. Intensity refers to the murmur's loudness.
7. To document a murmur's intensity, most health care professionals use a six-point graded scale, with 1 being the faintest intensity and 6 being the loudest. A grade 1 murmur is faint and is barely heard through the stethoscope. A grade 2 murmur is also faint but is usually heard as soon as the stethoscope is placed on the chest wall. A grade 3 murmur is easily heard and is described as moderately loud. A grade 4 murmur is loud and is usually associated with a palpable vibration known as a thrill. It also may radiate in the di-

rection of blood flow. A grade 5 murmur is loud enough to be heard with only an edge of the stethoscope touching the chest wall; it is almost always accompanied by a thrill and radiation. A grade 6 murmur is so loud that it can be heard with the stethoscope close to, but not touching, the chest wall; it is always accompanied by a thrill and it radiates to distant structures.

8. Duration, the length of time the murmur is heard during systole or diastole, may be described as long or short.

9. A murmur's pitch, or frequency, varies from high to low.

10. A murmur's quality is determined by the combination of frequencies that produces the sound. It is typically described as harsh, rough, musical, scratchy, squeaky, rumbling, or blowing.

11. A murmur's timing refers to when the murmur occurs in the cardiac cycle. This means that the onset, duration, and end of the murmur are described in relation to systole and diastole. Murmurs are further classified according to their timing within the phases of the cardiac cycle. For example, a murmur can be described as holosystolic (present throughout systole), or as early, mid-, or late systolic or diastolic.

12. Configuration refers to the shape of a murmur's sound as recorded on a phonocardiogram. The configuration is usually defined by changes in the murmur's intensity during systole or diastole and is determined by blood flow pressure gradients.

13. A crescendo murmur is one that gradually increases in intensity as the pressure gradient increases. A decrescendo murmur is one that gradually decreases in intensity as the pressure gradient decreases. A crescendo-decrescendo murmur first increases in intensity as the pressure gradient increases, then decreases in intensity as the pressure gradient decreases; it's also known as a diamond-shaped murmur. Finally, a plateau-shaped murmur is one that's equal in intensity throughout the murmur.

17 Systolic murmurs

1. Normally, as ventricular pressures rise at the beginning of systole, the mitral and tricuspid valves close. Then, for a brief time while the aortic and pulmonic valves are still closed during isovolumic contraction, ventricular pressures rise sharply. When the pressure

in both ventricles is high enough, the aortic and pulmonic valves open, and blood is ejected from the ventricles into the aorta and the pulmonary artery. Normally functioning valves facilitate this unidirectional blood flow. However, aortic or pulmonic outlet abnormalities may generate forward systolic ejection murmurs. When the mitral or tricuspid valve is involved, backward, or regurgitant, murmurs may be heard during systole.

2. During ventricular systole, the rapid ejection of blood from the ventricles causes turbulent blood flow, which produces an innocent systolic ejection murmur (SEM).

3. An SEM is usually heard best along the left sternal border and sometimes over the aortic and mitral areas. Its intensity is usually soft (less than a grade $\%$), and its duration is short. It has a medium pitch heard best with the diaphragm of the stethoscope. The quality of an SEM is variable. Its timing is early systolic; it ends well before a normal S_2 split. It is heard after the QRS complex in the ECG waveform. An SEM has a crescendo-decrescendo configuration.

4. An SEM's intensity can be increased by maneuvers that increase blood volume or ejection velocity, such as having the patient raise his legs from a recumbent position, exercise briefly, or cough a few times.

5. Right or left ventricular outflow obstructions may be supravalvular, valvular, or subvalvular. Regardless of location, the outflow obstruction causes turbulent blood flow, which produces a midsystolic ejection murmur. The murmur begins early in systole, after S_1 and the opening of the diseased pulmonic or aortic valve. It ends before the S_2 closure component of the diseased pulmonic or aortic valve. This murmur typically has a crescendo-decrescendo configuration that peaks in intensity in early, mid-, or late systole, depending on the severity of the obstruction.

6. The supravalvular pulmonic stenosis murmur is usually heard over much of the thorax. Its intensity and duration are variable. It has a medium pitch heard best with the diaphragm of the stethoscope and a harsh quality. Its timing is systolic: it begins after S_1 and ends before a normal S_2 split. In the ECG waveform, the murmur begins just after the QRS complex begins and ends just before the T wave ends. It has

a crescendo-decrescendo configuration that's occasionally continuous.

7. In mild pulmonic valvular stenosis, S_1 is normal. The murmur begins after S_1 with a right-sided pulmonic ejection sound (PES) as the pulmonic valve abruptly stops opening. The murmur intensifies after the PES, peaks in midsystole, and then begins to fade. It ends before S_2. The intensity of P_2 is normal.

In severe pulmonic valvular stenosis, the pressure gradient across the pulmonic valve increases. An increased pressure gradient causes the PES to be heard earlier; it may even fuse with S_1. Right ventricular ejection time is also prolonged. Consequently, the murmur has a longer crescendo and the intensity peaks later in systole. It continues throughout A_2 but ends before P_2. Prolonged right ventricular ejection time also causes a delayed P_2, creating a wide S_2 split. Usually, as the stenosis becomes more severe, the murmur's duration lengthens and its configuration becomes more asymmetrical. Consequently, P_2 is delayed even more and its intensity is decreased.

8. The pulmonic valvular stenosis murmur is heard best near the heart's base over the pulmonic area. It often radiates toward the left neck or the left shoulder. The murmur's intensity is usually soft, but it will become louder as the stenosis becomes more severe. Its duration is short, but this too will increase as the stenosis worsens. It has a medium pitch heard best with the diaphragm of the stethoscope and a harsh quality. The murmur's timing is midsystolic: It ends before a normal S_2 split. In the ECG waveform, it begins after the QRS complex and ends before the end of the T wave. It has a crescendo-decrescendo configuration. A mild pulmonic valvular stenosis murmur is shaped like a diamond; a severe pulmonic valvular stenosis murmur is shaped like a kite.

9. The subvalvular pulmonic stenosis murmur is usually heard best over the pulmonic area and over Erb's point; it often radiates toward the left side of the neck, the left shoulder, or both. Its intensity is usually soft but becomes louder as the stenosis worsens. Its duration, which is short, also increases as the stenosis worsens. The murmur has a medium pitch heard best with the diaphragm of the stethoscope; its quality is harsh. Its timing is midsystolic: It starts after S_1 and ends before a normal S_2 split. In the ECG waveform,

the murmur begins after the QRS complex and ends before the end of the T wave. This murmur is not initiated by a pulmonic ejection sound. It has a crescendo-decrescendo configuration.

10. The supravalvular aortic stenosis murmur is usually heard best near the heart's base over the right first intercostal space, over the aortic area, and over the suprasternal notch. It may radiate toward the right side of the neck, the right shoulder, or both. Its intensity, typically a grade ⅜ to ⅘, decreases in patients with left ventricular failure. Its duration increases as the stenosis worsens. It has a medium pitch that can be heard equally well with the diaphragm or bell of the stethoscope. The murmur has a rough quality. Its timing is midsystolic: It ends before a normal S_2 split. It is not associated with an aortic ejection sound. In the ECG waveform, it begins after the QRS complex and ends before the end of the T wave. The murmur has a crescendo-decrescendo configuration.

11. The aortic valvular stenosis murmur is usually heard best near the heart's base over the aortic area, over Erb's point, near the heart's apex over the mitral area, or over the suprasternal notch. The murmur may radiate toward the right side of the neck, the right shoulder, or both. A thrill may be palpable over the aortic area and neck. The intensity, typically a grade ⅜ to ⅘, decreases in patients with left ventricular failure. The murmur's duration increases as stenosis worsens.

    The aortic valvular stenosis murmur has a medium pitch heard equally well with the diaphragm or bell of the stethoscope. The murmur's quality is rough and may become harsher and louder as stenosis worsens. Its timing is midsystolic. An aortic ejection sound (AES), when present, is heard shortly after S_1; the AES is followed by the murmur, which ends before a normal S_2 split. In the ECG waveform, the murmur begins after the QRS complex and ends before the end of the T wave. It has a crescendo-decrescendo configuration.

12. A subvalvular aortic outflow obstruction may be caused by a congenital fibrous ring, or it may be acquired from hypertrophic cardiomyopathy.

13. The subvalvular aortic stenosis murmur is usually heard best near the heart's apex over the mitral and tricuspid areas. It does not usually radiate toward the base, right side of the neck, or the right shoulder. Its

intensity, typically a grade $\frac{3}{6}$ to $\frac{4}{6}$, will increase as stenosis worsens; its duration is variable. The murmur has a medium pitch heard equally well with the bell or diaphragm of the stethoscope. Its quality can be harsh or rough. This murmur's timing is midsystolic: It peaks in midsystole and ends before a normal S_2 split, a delayed A_2, or a paradoxical S_2 split. In the ECG waveform, it begins after the QRS complex and ends before the end of the T wave. The murmur has a crescendo-decrescendo configuration.

14. An abnormality of either the mitral or tricuspid valve may result in backward turbulent blood flow during systole. This means that blood moves in a direction opposite that of the normal unidirectional flow pattern. Blood regurgitates through a defective, incompetent mitral or tricuspid valve into the left or right atrium.

15. The tricuspid regurgitation murmur is usually heard best over the tricuspid area; in some patients, it is heard only during inspiration. The murmur may radiate to the right of the sternum. Its usually soft intensity may increase during deep inspiration. The murmur's duration is long. It has a high pitch heard best with the diaphragm of the stethoscope and a scratchy or blowing quality. The murmur's timing is systolic: It lasts from S_1 to P_2. In the ECG waveform, the murmur begins just after the QRS complex and ends after the T wave. It is holosystolic and plateau-shaped.

16. To enhance the murmur, have the patient breathe through his mouth slowly, quietly, and deeply while sitting or standing. Caution the patient not to hold his breath because this negates the maneuver's effect. The murmur is louder during inspiration. In some patients, this is the only time the murmur is audible.

17. An incompetent mitral valve causes backward blood flow through the incompetent mitral valve during systole. The increased resistance at the aortic valve facilitates regurgitation of blood through the incompetent mitral valve into the left atrium, producing the mitral regurgitation murmur.

18. The holosystolic mitral regurgitation murmur is usually heard best near the heart's apex over the mitral area. The sound may radiate to the axilla or posteriorly over the lung bases. Its intensity is variable and usually not affected by respiration; however, it may be somewhat diminished during inspiration. The murmur has a long duration. It has a medium to high

pitch heard best with the diaphragm of the stethoscope. The murmur may be accompanied by a systolic apical thrill. Its quality is blowing, and its timing is systolic — from S_1 to S_2. In the ECG waveform, it is heard from just after the QRS complex to the end of the T wave. The murmur is holosystolic and plateau-shaped.

19. The acute mitral regurgitation murmur is usually heard best near the heart's apex over the mitral area. Its intensity is usually loud (a grade ⁴⁄₆ to ⁶⁄₆ if the murmur results from rupture of the chordae tendineae). It is accompanied by a systolic thrill. The murmur's duration is long. It has a high pitch heard best with the diaphragm of the stethoscope and a quality that can be musical. Its timing is systolic: It begins with M_1 and ends with or before A_2. In the ECG waveform, the murmur begins just after the QRS complex and ends just after the T wave. It is holosystolic and wedge-shaped (the wedge shape has a steeper decrescendo configuration).

20. The mitral valve prolapse murmur is usually heard best near the heart's apex over the mitral area. Its intensity is usually soft (a grade ²⁄₆ to ³⁄₆), and its duration is short. It has a high pitch heard best with the diaphragm of the stethoscope. The murmur has a musical quality; when loud, it's sometimes described as a whoop or honk. Its timing is usually late systolic but can sometimes be holosystolic. In the ECG waveform, the murmur coincides with the T wave and ends just after the T wave. It has a crescendo or crescendo-decrescendo configuration.

21. Having the patient stand decreases left ventricular volume, which causes the mitral valve prolapse murmur to be heard earlier in systole, to be louder, and to last longer. Having the patient squat increases left ventricular volume, which causes the murmur to be heard later in systole.

18 Diastolic murmurs

1. At the end of ventricular systole and the beginning of diastole, the aortic and pulmonic valves close. During this time, the A_2–P_2 interval can usually be auscultated. After a brief period of isovolumic relaxation, the mitral and tricuspid valves open and blood flows from the atria into the ventricles. During this early

filling period, an S_3 can sometimes be heard in healthy individuals under age 40. Late in diastole, the atria contract, increasing blood flow into the ventricles. Occasionally, an S_4 can be heard during this late filling period. Except for these brief heart sounds, diastole is normally silent. When diastolic murmurs occur, they are heard between S_2 and S_1 or between the end of the T wave and the beginning of the QRS complex in the ECG waveform.

The regurgitation of blood through the aortic and pulmonic valves may cause diastolic murmurs. Because both valves close at the beginning of diastole, murmurs produced by dysfunctional aortic and pulmonic valves begin early in diastole, immediately after the affected valve closes.

Mitral and tricuspid valve stenosis and conditions that produce turbulent blood flow across normal mitral or tricuspid valves also cause diastolic murmurs. Because these valves open after a period of isovolumic relaxation, these murmurs are heard during mid-diastole.

2. The early diastolic aortic regurgitation murmur is usually heard best near the heart's base over the aortic and pulmonic areas, over Erb's point, and near the heart's apex over the mitral area. Because of its usually soft intensity, it is heard best in a quiet environment. The murmur can last throughout most of diastole. It has a high pitch heard best with the diaphragm of the stethoscope and a blowing or musical quality. Its timing is diastolic, beginning with A_2. In the ECG waveform, the murmur begins after the end of the T wave and ends just before the QRS complex. It has a decrescendo configuration.

3. This murmur can be enhanced by having the patient sit down, lean forward, and hold his breath after expiration or by maneuvers that increase aortic diastolic pressure, such as having the patient squat.

4. The Austin Flint murmur is usually heard best near the heart's apex over the mitral area. Its intensity is usually soft. It has a low pitch heard best with the bell of the stethoscope. The murmur has a rumbling quality. Its timing is confined to middiastole and presystole. It's heard just before the RS complex in the ECG waveform. The murmur has a presystolic crescendo configuration; its middiastolic component has a crescendo-decrescendo configuration.

5. The Graham Steell murmur secondary to pulmonary hypertension is usually heard best along the left sternal border over the third and fourth intercostal spaces. It is not transmitted to the right sternum. Its intensity is usually loud, and its duration is variable. The murmur has a high pitch heard best with the diaphragm of the stethoscope, and it has a blowing quality. Its timing is early diastolic, beginning with a loud P_2. Sometimes an ejection sound can be heard. The murmur is heard after the end of the T wave in the ECG waveform. It has a decrescendo configuration.

6. The Graham Steell murmur is intensified during inspiration.

7. The normal pressure pulmonic valve murmur is usually heard best along the left sternal border over the third and fourth intercostal spaces. It isn't transmitted to the right sternum. Its intensity is soft and its duration is brief. The murmur has a low pitch heard best with the bell of the stethoscope. It has a rumbling quality and its timing is early to middiastolic. It begins shortly after P_2 is heard. In the ECG waveform, it begins after the T wave and ends before the P wave. The murmur has a crescendo-decrescendo configuration.

8. The normal pressure pulmonic valve murmur is intensified during inspiration.

9. Scarring and calcification of the valve create a funnel-shaped opening between the left atrium and left ventricle. The mitral stenosis murmur starts with an opening snap (OS) after A_2 and isovolumic relaxation; this OS is an important diagnostic feature of mitral stenosis. The murmur is produced by rapid, turbulent blood flow through a rigid, narrowed mitral valve opening. Turbulence increases just before systole; this gives the murmur its characteristic presystolic crescendo.

10. The mitral stenosis murmur is usually heard best near the heart's apex over the mitral area. Its intensity and duration are variable. It has a low pitch heard best with the bell of the stethoscope and a rumbling quality that has been compared to thunder. The timing of a mitral stenosis murmur is diastolic: It begins after A_2 with an OS and ends with a loud M_1. However, stenosis severity affects the murmur's duration. In the ECG waveform, the murmur begins just after the T wave and ends during the QRS complex. It has

a crescendo-decrescendo configuration. In patients with normal sinus rhythm, the presystolic component has a crescendo configuration.

11. The mitral stenosis murmur is heard best with the patient in a partial left lateral recumbent position. It can be intensified by maneuvers that increase cardiac output, such as having the patient exercise for a few minutes, raise his legs from a recumbent position, or cough several times.

12. The tricuspid stenosis murmur is usually heard best over the tricuspid area. Its usually soft intensity increases during inspiration and fades or disappears during expiration. The murmur's duration is variable. It has a low pitch heard best with the bell of the stethoscope while the patient is in the partial left lateral recumbent position. The murmur has a rumbling quality. Its timing is mid- to late diastolic: It ends just before S_1. An opening snap may be heard. In the ECG waveform, the murmur begins just after the T wave and ends just before the QRS complex. In patients with normal sinus rhythm, it has a late diastolic crescendo or crescendo-decrescendo configuration.

19 Continuous murmurs

1. Continuous murmurs are generated by rapid blood flow through arteries or veins or by shunting. Shunting occurs when an abnormal communication is created between the high-pressure arterial system and the low-pressure venous system. The murmurs begin in systole and persist, without interruption, through S_2 into diastole.

2. The normal cervical venous hum is caused by rapid downward blood flow through the jugular veins in the lower part of the neck.

3. The cervical venous hum murmur is heard best over the right supraclavicular fossa when the patient is sitting and his head is turned to the left. It has a faint intensity that increases during diastole. The murmur has a long duration: It lasts throughout the cardiac cycle. Its high pitch is heard best with the diaphragm of the stethoscope. Its quality is soft and its timing is continuous. The hum is louder between S_2 and S_1. The murmur has a plateau shape in systole and a crescendo-decrescendo configuration in diastole.

4. The patent ductus arteriosus (PDA) murmur is heard best over the left first intercostal space, over the pulmonic area, and below the left clavicle. Its intensity is faint when the murmur is limited to this area. If the murmur is loud, the systolic component may be heard along the left sternal border and sometimes over the mitral area. A loud PDA murmur may radiate to the back between the scapulae. The PDA murmur has a long duration. Its intensity is variable, roughly correlating with the ductus size; typically, the murmur reaches maximum intensity late in systole and then fades during diastole. The PDA murmur has a high pitch heard equally well with the bell or diaphragm of the stethoscope. It has a rough, machinery-like quality, and its timing is continuous. It begins with, or shortly after, a normal S_1 and disappears just before the next S_1. Because the murmur peaks in late systole, S_2 may be difficult to hear. S_2 may be paradoxically split if left ventricular ejection time is prolonged. An S_3 may be heard over the mitral area. The murmur has a crescendo-decrescendo configuration.

5. Exercise can increase the intensity and duration of a PDA murmur.

6. To differentiate between a PDA murmur and a cervical venous hum murmur, remember that the hum is loudest above the clavicle, is usually heard better on the right, and can be obliterated by pressing on the jugular vein or placing the patient in a supine position. The venous hum is truly continuous and is usually louder during diastole.

20 Other auscultatory sounds

1. The aortic and mitral valves are most commonly replaced.

2. The four types of prosthetic valves used to replace human valves are the ball-in-cage, the tilting-disk, the bileaflet, and the porcine valves.

3. The murmur generated by an aortic ball-in-cage valve prosthesis is usually heard best near the apex over the mitral and aortic areas and along the left sternal border. Its intensity is usually loud and easy to hear, and its duration is variable. It has a medium pitch heard best with the diaphragm of the stethoscope. The murmur has a crunchy, harsh quality. Its timing is midsystolic. The interval between the aortic closing click and P_2 is similar to the normal A_2–P_2 interval, and it normally widens during inspiration. The murmur has a crescendo-decrescendo configuration.

4. Dysfunction of an aortic ball-in-cage valve prosthesis commonly causes the aortic opening click to become soft or absent; the aortic closing click may be absent too. A diastolic murmur and a long systolic ejection murmur may appear.

5. The murmur generated by an aortic tilting-disk valve prosthesis is usually heard best near the apex over the mitral and aortic areas and along the left sternal border. Its intensity is usually soft (grade ⅖), and its duration is short. It has a medium pitch heard best with the diaphragm of the stethoscope. The murmur has a rough or harsh quality. Its timing is systolic. The interval between the aortic closing click and P_2 is similar to the normal A_2–P_2 interval, and it widens during inspiration. The murmur has a crescendo-decrescendo configuration.

6. Dysfunction of an aortic tilting-disk valve prosthesis commonly causes some or all of the following changes: The aortic closing click may be absent, a diastolic murmur may be heard, a murmur that extends into the latter half of diastole may appear, or a longer systolic ejection murmur may appear.

7. The murmur generated by an aortic bileaflet valve prosthesis is usually heard best near the apex over the mitral and aortic areas and along the left sternal border. Its intensity is usually soft (grade ⅖), and its duration is short. It has a medium pitch heard best with the diaphragm of the stethoscope. The murmur has a rough or harsh quality, and its timing is systolic. The interval between the aortic closing click and P_2 is similar to the normal A_2–P_2 interval, and it widens during inspiration. The murmur has a crescendo-decrescendo configuration.

8. Dysfunction of the aortic bileaflet valve prosthesis may cause the aortic closing click to disappear, a diastolic murmur to appear, or both. A longer systolic ejection murmur also may appear.

9. The murmur generated by an aortic porcine valve prosthesis is usually heard best near the apex over the mitral and aortic areas and along the left sternal border. Its intensity is usually soft (grade ⅖), and its duration is short. It has a medium pitch heard best with the diaphragm of the stethoscope. The murmur

has a rough or harsh quality, and its timing is systolic. The interval between the aortic closing click and P_2 is similar to the normal A_2–P_2 interval, and it widens during inspiration. The murmur has a crescendo-decrescendo configuration.

10. Dysfunction of an aortic porcine valve prosthesis may cause the aortic closing click to be diminished, a diastolic murmur to appear, or both. A longer systolic ejection murmur also may appear.

11. When the systolic murmur generated by a mitral ball-in-cage valve prosthesis is audible, it is usually heard best near the apex over the mitral or tricuspid area. Its intensity is usually soft, and its duration is short. It has a medium pitch heard best with the diaphragm of the stethoscope. The murmur has a harsh quality, and its timing is systolic. A mitral opening click follows a normal S_2. The murmur has a crescendo-decrescendo configuration.

12. Dysfunction of a mitral ball-in-cage valve prosthesis may cause some or all of the following changes: The sounds normally associated with the valve may vary in intensity in a patient with normal sinus rhythm; a short interval between A_2 and the mitral opening click may occur, indicating high left atrial pressure; a holosystolic murmur may occur, indicating mitral regurgitation; or the intensity and duration of the diastolic murmur may change, indicating mitral obstruction.

13. The systolic murmur generated by a mitral tilting-disk valve prosthesis is usually heard best near the apex over the mitral area or, occasionally, over the tricuspid area. Its intensity is usually soft (grade ⅖). The murmur has a short duration and a high pitch heard best with the diaphragm of the stethoscope. It has a harsh quality and systolic timing. The murmur has a crescendo-decrescendo configuration.

14. Dysfunction of a mitral tilting-disk valve prosthesis may cause some or all of the-following changes: The mitral closing click may be absent, a new diastolic murmur may develop, a previously auscultated diastolic murmur may intensify, or a holosystolic mitral regurgitation murmur may appear.

15. The systolic murmur generated by a mitral bileaflet valve prosthesis is usually heard best near the apex over the mitral area or, occasionally, over the tricuspid area. Its intensity is usually soft (grade ⅖), and its du-

ration is short. It has a high pitch heard best with the diaphragm of the stethoscope. The murmur has a harsh quality and its timing is systolic. The mitral opening click, though rarely heard, follows a normal S_2. The murmur has a crescendo-decrescendo configuration.

16. Dysfunction of a mitral bileaflet valve prosthesis may cause a holosystolic murmur, a new diastolic murmur, or both to appear.

17. The systolic murmur generated by a mitral porcine valve prosthesis is usually heard best near the apex over the mitral area. Its intensity is usually soft (grade ²⁄₆ to ³⁄₆), and its duration is short. It has a medium pitch heard best with the diaphragm of the stethoscope and a harsh quality. Its timing is systolic. The murmur has a crescendo-decrescendo configuration.

18. Dysfunction of a mitral porcine valve prosthesis may cause a holosystolic mitral regurgitation murmur, a diastolic rumble associated with mitral stenosis, or both to appear.

19. When inflamed pericardial surfaces rub together, they produce characteristic high-pitched friction noises known as pericardial friction rubs.

20. A pericardial friction rub is usually heard best, and is sometimes palpable, over the tricuspid and xyphoid areas. It is usually loud and may get louder during inspiration. The rub has a high pitch heard best with the diaphragm of the stethoscope, and it has a grating or scratchy quality. It is usually heard during each cardiac cycle. It has a systolic component and an early and late diastolic component. The diastolic component may last for only a few hours.

21. You can easily differentiate a pericardial friction rub from a pleural friction rub by having the patient hold his breath. When he does so, a pericardial friction rub will persist, but a pleural friction rub will become inaudible.

22. Heart movements can displace air that is present in the mediastinum; this displacement produces crunchy noises — known as mediastinal crunch — that may occur randomly or in a consistent pattern.

23. The noises produced by mediastinal crunch are usually heard best near the apex over the mitral area and along the left sternal border with the patient in the partial left lateral recumbent position. The noises have a crunching quality, which may become louder during inspiration.

Selected references

Braunwald, E. *Heart Disease: Textbook of Cardiovascular Medicine,* 5th ed. Philadelphia: W.B. Saunders Co., 1997.

Burton, G., et al., eds. *Respiratory Care: A Guide to Clinical Practice,* 4th ed. Philadelphia: Lippincott-Raven Pubs., 1997.

Cahalin, L. "Auscultation of the Heart: A Cursory Review of Basic Principles and Practice Skills," *Cardiopulmonary Physical Therapy Journal* 8(2):8-11, Spring 1997.

Diseases, 2nd ed. Springhouse, Pa.: Springhouse Corp., 1997.

ECG Interpretation Made Incredibly Easy! Springhouse, Pa.: Springhouse Corp., 1997.

Erickson, B. *Heart Sounds and Murmurs: A Practical Guide,* 3rd ed. St. Louis: Mosby–Year Book, Inc., 1997.

Faucia, S., et al., eds. *Harrison's Principles of Internal Medicine,* 14th ed. New York: McGraw Hill Book Co., 1998.

Hudak, C.M., and Gallo, B.M. *Critical Care Nursing: A Holistic Approach,* 7th ed. Philadelphia: Lippincott-Raven Pubs., 1998.

Kirton, C. "Assessing S_3 and S_4 Heart Sounds," *Nursing97* 27(7):52-53, July 1997.

O'Hanlon-Nichols, T. "Basic Assessment Series: The Adult Cardiovascular System," *AJN* 97(12):34-40, December 1997.

Owen, A. "Respiratory Assessment Revisited," *Nursing98* 28(4):48-49, April 1998.

Petty, T.L. *The 1997 Yearbook of Pulmonary Disease.* St. Louis: Mosby–Year Book, Inc., 1997.

Professional Guide to Diseases, 6th ed. Springhouse, Pa.: Springhouse Corp., 1998.

Professional Guide to Signs and Symptoms, 2nd ed. Springhouse, Pa.: Springhouse Corp., 1997.

Rosse, C., and Gaddum-Rosse, P. *Hollinshead's Textbook of Anatomy.* Philadelphia: Lippincott-Raven Pubs., 1997.

Textbook of Advanced Cardiac Life Support. Dallas: American Heart Association, 1998.

Turner, P., et al., "Care of the Patient Requiring Mechanical Ventilation," *Medical Surgical Nursing* 6(2):68-73, 76-78, 94, April 1997.

Glossary

A$_2$ Aortic component of S$_2$.

Accessory muscles of respiration   Muscles involved in labored, or forceful, breathing. They include the sternocleidomastoid, scalene, trapezius, and rhomboid muscles.

Acoustical mismatch   Phenomenon in which sounds transmitted through two different media, such as air and tissue, are diminished in intensity or blocked.

Acute pulmonary hypertension   Sudden increased pressure within the pulmonary circulation (above 30 mm Hg systolic and 12 mm Hg diastolic).

Adult respiratory distress syndrome   Disease with numerous etiologies that's characterized by interstitial and alveolar edema and progressive hypoxemia; also known as *shock lung* or *posttraumatic lung*.

Adventitious sound   An acquired (usually) abnormal sound superimposed over normal or abnormal breath sounds.

AES   Aortic ejection sound.

Alveolar-capillary membrane   Cell membrane across which oxygen and carbon dioxide must diffuse for respiration to occur.

Alveolar duct   Portion of the airway that is completely lined with alveoli.

Alveolus   One of the millions of very small, saclike lung structures where oxygen–carbon dioxide exchange occurs.

Amplitude   Magnitude or intensity of a sound.

Anatomic dead space   Air that remains in the conducting airways during each breath. This air isn't involved in oxygen–carbon dioxide exchange.

Antigen   Substance or material foreign to the body that causes a reaction leading to the formation of antibodies.

Aortic ejection sound   Opening sound of a stenotic aortic valve. It follows S$_1$ early in ventricular systole and appears just after the QRS complex on the ECG.

Aortic regurgitation   Abnormal condition of turbulent backward blood flow through the aortic valve into the left ventricle during diastole.

Aortic stenosis   Narrowing or constriction of the aortic orifice or of the aorta itself.

Aortic valve Membranous folds that prevent blood reflux from the aorta into the left ventricle.

Aortic valvular stenosis Constriction of or damage to the aortic valve that restricts forward blood flow from the left ventricle to the aorta during systole.

ARDS Adult respiratory distress syndrome.

Arteriovenous shunt Direct passage of blood from arteries to veins, bypassing the capillary bed. This can refer to a physiologic response of the body or to an abnormal condition sometimes caused by trauma or surgery.

Asbestosis Lung disease characterized by pulmonary inflammation and fibrosis; caused by prolonged asbestos exposure.

Ascending aortic aneurysm Dilation of the initial part of the aorta.

Aspiration Act of inhaling; usually refers to the breathing in of foreign materials.

Asthma Disease characterized by bronchoconstriction, bronchospasm, airway edema, and excess mucus production, which lead to obstructed airflow, wheezing, and shortness of breath.

Atelectasis Incomplete expansion of the lung tissue usually caused by pressure from exudate, fluid, tumor, or an obstructed airway; may involve a lung segment or an entire lobe.

Atrial septal defect Imperfection, failure to develop fully, or absence of the dividing wall between the heart's atria.

Atrioventricular node Small mass of specialized cardiac tissue, located in the lower portion of the right atrium near the septum, that transmits electrical impulses from the sinoatrial node to the bundle of His.

Atrioventricular valves Valves between the atria and the ventricles — specifically, the tricuspid valve of the heart's right side and the mitral valve of the heart's left side.

Attenuation Decrease in the intensity or loudness of a breath sound.

Auscultation Act of listening to sounds made by the body; usually performed with a stethoscope.

Austin Flint murmur Heart sound generated by turbulent blood flow across the mitral valve; caused by aortic regurgitation, which closes the mitral leaflets.

AV   Atrioventricular.

Axillary fold   One of two anatomic landmarks anterior and posterior to the armpit, formed by the normal contour of the skin over the pectoralis major muscle anteriorly and the latissimus dorsi muscle posteriorly.

Ball-in-cage valve   Prosthetic heart valve characterized by a caged ball that moves with ventricular pressure to open and close the valvular opening.

Bell   Cup-shaped portion of the stethoscope that is best suited for listening to low-pitched sounds.

Bifurcate   To divide into two branches.

Bileaflet valve   Prosthetic heart valve characterized by two small wings that control blood flow.

Binaural headpiece   Stethoscope headpiece that supplies sounds to both ears simultaneously.

Blowing   Term used to describe a continuous murmur sound like the sound of air passing through pursed lips.

Booming   Term used to describe a deep, resonant heart sound that is sudden and percussive.

Bronchial circulation   Oxygenated blood that arises from the aorta or subclavicular artery and supplies the tracheobronchial tree with oxygen and nutrients.

Bronchial gland   One of the glands secreting mucus and serous liquid in the tracheobronchial tree. These glands are most numerous in the medium-sized bronchi and are the main source of bronchial secretions.

Bronchiectasis   Irreversible dilation of the bronchi characterized by chronic cough and sputum production and by fibrosed and atelectatic lung tissue surrounding the affected airways.

Bronchophony   Voice sound auscultated over the chest wall that reveals exaggerated vocal resonance.

Bronchospasm   Smooth muscle contraction within the airway walls, which leads to airway narrowing and reduced airflow.

Bronchovesicular breath sound   Normal breath sound auscultated between the mainstem bronchi and lung periphery; also known as a *transitional breath sound*.

Bundle of His   Small band of specialized cardiac muscle fibers that relay the atrial electrical impulses to the ventricles.

Capacitance   Heart's or vasculature's ability to receive or admit blood volume and the decreased resistance that accompanies it.

Capillary hydrostatic pressure   Fluid pressure within the capillary system, which, when elevated, leads to fluid extravasation out of the capillary system into the interstitium.

Cardiac cycle   Sequence of events (systole and diastole) that enables the heart to receive and pump blood.

Cardiac output   Quantity of oxygenated blood pumped through the body by the heart, usually expressed in liters per minute.

Cardiac tamponade   Heart compression caused by effusion or collection of fluid in the pericardium, resulting in decreased cardiac output.

Cervical venous hum murmur   Murmur caused by rapid downward blood flow through the jugular veins in the lower part of the neck.

Chordae tendineae   Tendinous cords that connect each cusp of the two atrioventricular valves to appropriate papillary muscles in the ventricles.

Chronic bronchitis   Disease characterized by chronic cough and sputum production that persists over a long period of time.

Chronic obstructive pulmonary disease   Chronic lung disease characterized by obstructed bronchial airflow or exhalation. Chronic bronchitis, emphysema, and asthma are types of obstructive lung disease.

Cilia   Motile, whiplike extensions from cell surfaces. Ciliated columnar epithelial cells line the walls of the tracheobronchial tree.

Click   Short heart sound; also, another term for a midsystolic sound that occurs when a prolapsed mitral valve's leaflet and chordae tendineae tense.

Click-murmur syndrome   Condition in which a click is followed by a murmur, as in mitral valve prolapse syndrome.

Closing click   Heart sound generated by valve closure. Closing clicks are heard with all prosthetic valves regardless of their type or position.

CM   Continuous murmur.

Coarctation of the aorta   Localized aortic malformation characterized by deformity of the aortic media and causing severe narrowing of the aortic lumen.

Compliance   Tissue's or organ's ability to yield to pressure without disruption; often used to describe the distensibility of an air- or fluid-filled organ, such as the heart or lungs.

Conchae   Shell-shaped turbinate bones in the nasal cavity that stimulate turbulent airflow within the nasal passages. The dense mucus and capillary beds that line the turbinates' surface encourage warming and humidification of inspired air.

Conducting airway   One of the airways beginning at the nose and ending at the terminal bronchioles. These airways are responsible for transporting air during breathing but are not involved in oxygen — carbon dioxide exchange.

Conduction system   Specialized cardiac cells and fibers that relay the electrical impulses, stimulating the heart muscle to contract.

Configuration   Shape of a murmur's sound as recorded on a phonocardiogram; one of the characteristics used to describe murmurs.

Congestion   Abnormal accumulation of fluid or blood in an organ or organ part.

Consolidation   Inflammatory solidification of lung tissue.

Constrictive pericarditis   Inflammation of the pericardium that leads to thickening and possible calcification of that sac, resulting in impaired diastolic filling, inflow stasis, or a constrictive effect.

Continuous murmur   Murmur that begins in systole and persists, without interruption, through S_2 into diastole.

Contractile cell   One of the myocardial cells that contract to start systole. These cells depolarize and repolarize by means of ion flow.

Contralateral   Referring to the opposite side or opposing symmetrical structure.

COPD   Chronic obstructive pulmonary disease.

Cor pulmonale   Heart disease caused by pulmonary hypertension secondary to disease of the lung or its blood vessels, with hypertrophy of the right ventricle.

Crackle   Short, explosive or popping sound usually heard during inspiration; described as *coarse* (loud and low in pitch) or *fine* (less intense and high in pitch); formerly known as a *rale*.

Crepitation   Crackling sound that resembles the sound made by rubbing hair between two fingers.

Crescendo   Term used to describe the configuration of a murmur that increases in intensity.

Crescendo-decrescendo   Term used to describe the configuration of a murmur that rises in intensity and then fades away.

Cusp   One of the triangular segments of a cardiac valve or one of the semilunar segments of the aortic or pulmonary valve.

Damped   Diminished sound intensity or amplitude; term used to describe sounds.

Decrescendo   Term used to describe the configuration of a murmur that decreases in intensity.

Dependent lung regions   Lowest lung regions (the lung bases when the patient is upright).

Depolarization   Movement of sodium ions into a contractile cell, creating a positive charge inside the cell.

Diamond-shaped murmur   Crescendo-decrescendo murmur.

Diaphragm   Primary muscle of respiration, which separates the thoracic and abdominal cavities; also the part of the stethoscope used to auscultate for high-pitched sounds.

Diastole   Expansion of the ventricles occurring in the interval between S_2 and S_1. The heart muscle, relaxing, fills with blood during this part of the cardiac cycle.

Diffuse   Widely distributed; not localized.

Dilation of pulmonic valve ring   Expansion of a valve aperture. A dilated pulmonic valve can contribute to a Graham Steell murmur.

Distribution of ventilation   Movement or circulation of air to specific lung regions during breathing.

DM   Diastolic murmur.

Dull percussion note   Deadened, or nonresonant, sound heard when an organ or body part is percussed.

Duration   Length of time a heart or breath sound is heard; one of the six characteristics used to describe heart sounds.

Dynamic airway compression   Narrowing of the airways during expiration caused by properties of intrapleural pressure, radial traction exerted by lung parenchyma, and the loss of elastic recoil within the lung.

Dynamic obstruction   Blocked outflow from one of the heart's chambers that can be demonstrated only during myocardial contraction or systole.

Dyspnea   Difficult or labored breathing.

Early diastolic aortic regurgitation   Blood backflow from the aorta that occurs early in diastole, when the ventricle is resting and filling with oxygenated blood.

ECG   Electrocardiogram.

Ectopic beats   Arrhythmic heartbeats arising from places other than the heart's normal pacemaker, the sinoatrial node.

Edema   Excessive accumulation of fluid in intercellular tissue spaces of the body.

Egophony   Voice sound that has a nasal or bleating quality when auscultated over the chest wall.

Ejection sound   Sound caused by the opening of a stenotic aortic or pulmonic valve, usually occurring early in systole.

Ejection velocity   Measure of the speed of blood flow.

Elastic recoil   Spontaneous contraction of lung parenchyma that occurs during expiration and that helps move air out of the lungs.

Elastic tension   Support and traction exerted on the airways because of the natural elastic recoil properties of the surrounding lung parenchyma.

Epicardial pacing   Regulation of the rate of heart muscle contraction by an artificial cardiac pacemaker stimulating the heart through electrical leads attached to the heart surface.

Epiglottis   Small elastic cartilage attached at the larynx that covers the opening to the trachea during swallowing.

Equal pressure point   Point in the airways where intrapulmonary and intrapleural pressures are equal.

Erb's point   Third intercostal space, left sternal border (3LSB).

ES   Ejection sound.

Exudate   Inflammatory fluid leaked from body cells or tissues.

Fibrosis Abnormal formation of fibrous connective tissue that is usually occurs as a reparative or reactive process within a tissue or organ.

5LMCL Fifth intercostal space, left midclavicular line (mitral area).

5LSB Fifth intercostal space, left sternal border (tricuspid area).

FRC Functional residual capacity.

Frequency Pitch of a breath sound measured in hertz.

Functional murmur Benign murmur that does not impair heart activity.

Gallop rhythm The S_1, S_2, S_3 sequence; the S_4, S_1, S_2 sequence; or both.

Gas exchange surface Alveolar capillary surface that is actively involved in diffusing oxygen and carbon dioxide.

Graham Steell murmur Pulmonic regurgitation murmur caused by pulmonic hypertension and pulmonic valve ring dilation.

Heart failure Clinical syndrome caused by left or right heart failure. Left heart failure results in pulmonary edema and breathlessness. Right heart failure results in liver congestion, increased venous pressure, and peripheral edema.

Hemidiaphragm One-half of the diaphragm (either the right or left side).

High-output condition Physiologic state that causes or results in increased cardiac output.

Hila Medial lung aspects where the bronchi, nerves, and vessels enter and leave.

Holodiastolic Pertaining to the entire diastole; used to describe a murmur that persists throughout diastole.

Holosystolic Pertaining to the entire systole; used to describe a murmur that persists throughout systole.

Holosystolic mitral regurgitation Blood backflow that is caused by an incompetent mitral valve and that can be heard throughout systole.

Hyperinflation Overinflation of the lung that occurs with air trapping in obstructive lung diseases such as emphysema.

Hypertrophic cardiomyopathy   Narrowing or constriction of the left ventricle's subaortic region caused by tissue enlargement in that area; also known as idiopathic hypertrophic subaortic stenosis. This condition can be a cause of subvalvular aortic stenosis.

Hypertrophy   Enlargement or overgrowth of an organ, or part of an organ, caused by an increase in the size of its constituent cells.

Hypoxemia   Abnormally low oxygen tension in arterial blood.

Hz   Hertz.

I:E ratio   Inspiratory-expiratory ratio.

Idiopathic   Of unknown cause.

Impedance matching   Similar acoustical characteristics of two organs or types of tissue that allow effective sound transmission.

Incompetent valve   Heart valve that cannot perform its functions because of congenital defects, disease, or trauma.

Infective endocarditis   Inflammation of the endocardium caused by infection with microorganisms (bacteria or fungi); primarily affects the heart valves.

Inferior vena cava   Venous trunk for the lower extremities and the pelvic and abdominal viscera.

Inspiratory-expiratory (I:E) ratio   Numerical expression of the duration of inspiration in relation to the duration of expiration.

Intensity   Degree of loudness; one of the six characteristics used to describe heart sounds.

Intercostal muscle   One of the muscles found between the ribs. Internal and external intercostal muscles help stabilize and expand or lower the rib cage with ventilation.

Internodal pathway   One of the fibers connecting the small masses of tissue that transmit the electrical impulses setting the heart's rate and rhythm.

Interstitial fibrosis   Abnormal formation of fibrous tissue that occurs as a reparative or reactive process within the alveolar septa and interstitial areas of the lungs.

Interstitium   Small gap in an organ or a tissue; in lung parenchyma, the space between the alveolar and capillary membranes.

Interventricular septum   Dividing wall between the heart's ventricles.

Intrapleural pressure   Relative pressure that occurs between the pleurae. Negative pressure occurs during inspiration; positive pressure occurs during expiration.

Intrapulmonary pressure   Pressure within the lung. Negative pressure causes air to flow inward; positive pressure causes air to move outward.

Isovolumic contraction   Initial period in early systole when the atrioventricular and semilunar valves are closed and intraventricular pressures rise, but blood has not yet been ejected from the ventricles.

Isovolumic relaxation   Brief period in early diastole when the atrioventricular and semilunar valves are closed, just before the atrioventricular valves open and passive filling of the ventricles begins.

Laminar airflow   Orderly, linear airflow.

Larynx   Cartilaginous organ located between the pharynx and the trachea that houses the vocal cords and allows for voice production.

Leaflet   Structure resembling a small leaf, especially a heart valve's cusps.

Left atrial shunt   Small amount of deoxygenated blood that returns to the left atrium; normally, this is venous return from bronchial circulation.

Left bundle-branch block   Interrupted conduction through the fiber that activates the left ventricle, resulting in a prolonged QRS complex.

Left lateral recumbent position   Position that brings the heart's apex closer to the chest wall for auscultation. The patient lies on his left side, with his right knee and thigh drawn up to his chest.

Left mainstem bronchus   One of two main branches extending from the trachea that supplies air to the left lung. It leaves the trachea at a sharper angle than the right mainstem bronchus and passes under the aortic arch before entering the lung.

Left ventricular decompensation   Failure of the left ventricle's myocardium to contract and maintain adequate cardiac output.

Left ventricular heart failure Inability of the left ventricle to pump blood adequately, causing decreased cardiac output, which results in pulmonary congestion and edema.

Left ventricular hypertrophy Enlargement of the left ventricle's myocardium, which can result in reduced or abnormal ventricular functioning.

Left ventricular outflow obstruction Stenosis or other blockage preventing flow of oxygenated blood from the left ventricle into the aorta.

Left ventricular pressure overload Increased pressure within the left ventricle that impairs its ability to function normally; often caused by excessively elevated systemic blood pressure.

Left ventricular volume overload Excessive volume within the left ventricle that causes it to become distended and impairs its ability to function normally.

Lobar Referring to or involving any lung lobe.

Location Site at which a breath sound can be auscultated.

Lower airway *See* Tracheobronchial tree.

Low-pitched wheeze Continuous, low-pitched sound that resembles snoring; previously classified as a *sonorous bronchus* or a *sonorous rale*.

M_1 Mitral component of S_1.

Macrophage Large ameboid, mononuclear cell that acts as a defense mechanism against infection; one of three cell types lining the alveoli.

Mainstem bronchi breath sound Harsh, tubular (hollow) breath sound heard over a mainstem bronchus.

Mast cell Connective tissue cell whose specific physiologic function remains unknown. The secretory mast cells on the surface of the large airways may be stimulated or affected by drugs, hormones, antigens, or other messenger cells to precipitate or control bronchoconstriction.

Mean airflow velocity Air flow rates occurring within an airway during the middle part of exhalation.

Mechanical ventilation Breathing that is assisted or controlled by a ventilator.

Mediastinal crunch Heart sound created by heart movement against air in the mediastinum.

Mediastinum   Tissues separating the two lungs, between the sternum and the vertebral column and from the thoracic inlet to the diaphragm. It contains the heart and its vessels, the trachea, esophagus, thymus, lymph nodes, and other organs and tissues.

Middiastolic aortic regurgitation   Turbulent backward blood flow through the aorta into the left ventricle occurring midway between S_2 and S_1.

Middiastolic click   Click heard midway between S_2 and S_1 in the cardiac cycle; usually associated with a stenotic or rigid atrioventricular valve.

Midsystolic ejection murmur   Crisp, high frequency sound resulting from a stenotic aortic or pulmonic valve opening in systole.

Mitral regurgitation   Turbulent backward blood flow from the left ventricle into the left atrium caused by the mitral valve's inability to close completely.

Mitral stenosis   Mitral valve narrowing or constriction.

Mitral valve   Tissue folds that, when closed, prevent blood flow from the left ventricle to the left atrium; also called the bicuspid valve.

Mitral valve prolapse   Mitral valve bulging from the proper position back toward the left atrium during systole.

Monophonic   Having one distinct musical sound or tone; used to describe selected wheezes.

MSC   Midsystolic click.

Mucus   Serous, watery liquid secreted by bronchial glands and goblet cells within the airways.

Murmur   Sound heard during auscultation that results from vibrations produced by blood moving within the heart and adjacent blood vessels; may be benign or abnormal.

Myocardial infarction   Tissue death in the heart's muscle; usually caused by inadequate coronary artery perfusion.

Myocardium   Heart wall, comprised of cardiac muscle tissue.

Nonejection click   Click caused by a valve that is not associated with movement of blood through or across the valve; often used to describe the click of mitral valve prolapse.

Normal breath sound   Sound auscultated over chest wall areas of a healthy person.

Normal sinus rhythm Normal physiologic heart rhythm originating in the sinoatrial node; usually considered to be 60 to 100 beats per minute.

O_2–CO_2 exchange Oxygen–carbon dioxide exchange

Opening click Opening sound created by some prosthetic heart valves or by a diseased valve.

Opening snap Sound created by mitral valve leaflets that have become stenotic or abnormally narrowed but that are still somewhat mobile.

Oscillation Vibration, fluctuation.

OS Opening snap.

P_2 Pulmonic component of S_2.

Papillary muscle Muscular protrusion, or projection, in the ventricles that attaches to and regulates the atrioventricular valves by way of the chordae tendineae.

Parasympathetic nervous system Part of the involuntary nervous system that supplies innervation to the internal organs. The hormone mediator is acetylcholine. The vagus nerve is a parasympathetic nerve that innervates the airways and, when stimulated, causes smooth muscle contraction, cough, and mucus discharge from the bronchial glands.

Parenchyma Functioning cells of an organ that distinguish or determine the primary organ function.

Patent ductus arteriosus Abnormal channel connecting the pulmonary artery to the descending aorta; results in arterial blood recirculation through the lungs.

PCG Phonocardiogram.

PDA Patent ductus arteriosus.

PEEP Positive end-expiratory pressure.

Perfusion Blood flow to or through an organ or tissue supplied by the blood vessels.

Pericardial fluid Fluid in the space between the visceral and parietal layers of the pericardium.

Pericardial friction rub Characteristic high-pitched friction noise created by inflamed pericardial surfaces rubbing together.

Pericardial knock S_3 associated with constrictive pericarditis.

Pericarditis Inflammation of the pericardium.

Pericardium   Two-layer fibrous sac that surrounds the heart and the roots of the great vessels.

Peripheral   Toward the outer boundary or perimeter; not central.

Peripheral vascular resistance   Resistance to the passage of blood through the small blood vessels, especially the arterioles, caused by friction between the blood and the blood vessel wall.

PES   Pulmonic ejection sound.

Pharynx   Musculomembranous passage between the posterior nares and the larynx and esophagus; also referred to as the throat. It serves as a joint conduit for food and air.

Phonation   Production of vocal sounds.

Phonocardiogram   Graphic record of heart sounds and murmurs, including pulse tracings, produced by phonocardiography.

Physiologic S_3 S_3 that is not associated with an abnormal condition; often found in young individuals.

Pitch   A tone's vibration or frequency, measured in cycles per second as sound amplitude; subjectively described as high, medium, or low.

Plateau-shaped murmur   Murmur in which intensity is the same, or flat, throughout its duration.

Pleurae   Thin, serous membranes that surround the lungs (visceral pleura) and line the thoracic cavity's inner walls (parietal pleura).

Pleural crackle   Loud, grating sound caused by inflamed or damaged pleurae; also called *pleural friction rub*.

Pleural effusion   Abnormal accumulation of fluid between visceral and parietal pleurae.

Pleural friction rub   Sound created by friction between the parietal and visceral pleurae surrounding the lungs; similar to a pericardial friction rub.

PMI   Point of maximum impulse.

Pneumonia   Inflammation of the lung parenchyma.

Pneumothorax   Accumulation of air within the pleural cavity.

Point of maximum impulse   Chest wall site where the heartbeat can be seen or felt most strongly; often located over the heart's apex.

Polyphonic   Having multiple distinct musical sounds or tones; used to describe selected wheezes.

Porcine valve   Prosthetic heart valve made from swine products.

Positive end-expiratory pressure   Application of positive pressure to exhalation during mechanical ventilation; used to help reexpand atelectatic areas and improve oxygenation.

Pressure gradient   Difference in pressure between two regions.

PR interval   Time between atrial contraction and ventricular contraction, as recorded on the ECG. The PR interval begins at the onset of the P wave and lasts until the onset of the QRS complex.

Prosthetic valve   Artificial heart valve replacing a nonfunctional valve. Ball-in-cage, bileaflet, porcine, and tilting-disk are four kinds of prosthetic heart valves.

Pulmonary artery   Blood vessel leading from the right ventricle to the lungs.

Pulmonary artery dilation   Expansion or stretching of the pulmonary artery beyond its normal dimensions.

Pulmonary circulation   Blood pumped by the right ventricle into the pulmonary artery that circulates through the pulmonary capillary beds, where gas exchange occurs. The oxygenated blood is carried to the left atrium via the pulmonary veins.

Pulmonary edema   Excessive accumulation of fluid within the lung.

Pulmonary hypertension   Increased blood pressure within the pulmonary circulation.

Pulmonary vein   One of four veins that return oxygenated blood from the lungs to the heart's left atrium.

Pulmonic ejection sound   High-pitched click commonly created by the opening of a stenotic pulmonic valve. It is the only right-sided heart sound whose intensity increases during expiration and decreases during inspiration.

Pulmonic regurgitation   Abnormal condition of backward blood flow across the pulmonic valve during diastole.

Pulmonic stenosis   Narrowing or constriction of the pulmonic valve or the region just above or below the valve.

Pulmonic valvular stenosis Narrowing or constriction of the pulmonic valve.

Purkinje fibers Modified cardiac muscle cells found beneath the endocardium. They are part of the heart's electrical impulse-conducting system.

P wave Part of the ECG tracing that represents atrial depolarization.

QRS complex ECG waves representing the spread of electrical impulses from the bundle branches to the ventricular muscle. The QRS complex corresponds to ventricular depolarization.

Quality Heart sound characteristic determined by a combination of the sound's frequencies; one of six characteristics used to describe heart sounds. A sound's quality may be described as sharp, dull, booming, snapping, blowing, harsh, or musical.

Radiation Spread of a heart sound beyond its area of origin.

Rale *See* Crackle.

Regurgitant murmur Sound created by turbulent backward blood flow through an incompetent heart valve.

Repolarization Movement of calcium ions into the cell and potassium ions out of the cell, followed by the extrusion of sodium and calcium ions from the cell and the restoration of potassium ions into the cell by the sodium-potassium pump.

Resistance Force that hinders motion; hindrance or impedance.

Resonance Sound quality produced by percussing structures or cavities that radiate sound vibrations and energy.

Respiratory cycle One complete cycle of inspiration and expiration.

Rheumatic heart disease Valvular abnormalities that are a sequela of rheumatic fever; most commonly, mitral, tricuspid, or aortic stenosis and insufficiency.

Rhonchus *See* Low-pitched wheeze.

Right bundle-branch block Interrupted conduction through the fiber that activates the right ventricle, resulting in a prolonged QRS complex.

Right mainstem bronchus   One of two main branches extending from the trachea that supplies air to the right lung. It leaves the trachea at a less-acute angle than the left mainstem bronchus.

Right-sided S_3   Heart sound caused by a noncompliant right ventricle and high right atrial pressure. It is heard in patients with cor pulmonale, pulmonary embolism, right ventricular failure secondary to mitral stenosis with left-sided heart failure or pulmonary hypertension, and severe tricuspid insufficiency.

Right-sided S_4 S_4 generated in the right ventricle; often heard in conditions that create pressures greater than 100 mm Hg in that ventricle. It may accompany such conditions as pulmonic stenosis, pulmonary hypertension, or sudden tricuspid regurgitation.

Right ventricular failure   Inability of the right ventricle to continue functioning properly.

Right ventricular outflow obstruction   Stenosis, embolus, or other blockage preventing flow of deoxygenated blood from the right ventricle into the pulmonary artery.

S_1   First heart sound.

S_2   Second heart sound.

S_3   Third heart sound; created by vibrations caused by the rapid, passive filling of the ventricles. S_3 is abnormal in adults over age 40.

S_4   Fourth heart sound; generated by stretching and filling of a ventricle during late diastole; associated with atrial contraction.

SA   Sinoatrial.

Sarcoidosis   Granulomatous lung disease of unknown origin that may cause pulmonary fibrosis.

Scapula   Triangular flat bone that makes up part of the shoulder girdle; also known as the *shoulder blade*.

Segmental bronchus   Airway that branches from a lobar bronchus and conducts air to a lung segment.

SEM   Systolic ejection murmur (also referred to as SM).

Semilunar valves   Heart valves between the ventricles and the pulmonary artery and aorta.

Serous   Having a watery consistency.

Shunting   Abnormal communication between the high-pressure arterial system and the low-pressure venous system.

Silent chest   Absence of breath sounds during auscultation; usually associated with severe bronchospasm and insufficient airflow to produce sounds.

Sinoatrial node   Small mass of tissue at the junction of the superior vena cava and the right atrium, which triggers the electrical impulses that begin the cardiac cycle.

SM   Systolic murmur (also referred to as SEM).

Snap   Short, sharp heart sound associated with sudden closing or opening of a heart valve.

Status asthmaticus   Severe asthma that is resistant to treatment; characterized by respiratory insufficiency or failure, wheezing, and severe dyspnea.

Stenosis   Narrowing or constriction of a bodily passage; specifically, a heart valve or region around the outflow tract of any of the heart's chambers, or an airway.

Sternal border   Auscultatory area along and to either side of the sternum.

Stethoscope   Instrument used in auscultation; usually consists of a diaphragm and a bell, which are connected to one or two tubes leading to a binaural headpiece and earpieces.

Stridor   Noisy, high-pitched sound that can usually be heard at a distance from the patient; caused by laryngeal spasm and mucosal swelling, which contract the vocal cords and narrow the airway.

Stroke volume   Amount of blood pumped during each ventricular contraction.

Subcutaneous emphysema   Presence of air or gas in the tissues beneath the skin.

Subvalvular aortic stenosis murmur   Murmur caused by a left ventricular outflow obstruction below the aortic valve.

Subvalvular pulmonic stenosis   Narrowing or constriction of the region below the pulmonic valve.

Subvalvular pulmonic stenosis murmur   Murmur caused by a right ventricular outflow obstruction below the pulmonic valve.

Summation gallop S_4 that occurs simultaneously with S_3, thus sounding louder.

Superior vena cava   Major vein that drains blood from the upper half of the body, beginning below the right costal cartilage and continuing to the right atrium.

Supine   Lying on the back, face up.

Supravalvular aortic stenosis murmur   Murmur caused by left ventricular outflow obstruction above the aortic valve.

Supravalvular pulmonic stenosis   Narrowing or constriction of the region above the pulmonic valve.

Supravalvular pulmonic stenosis murmur   Murmur caused by a right ventricular outflow obstruction above the pulmonic valve.

Surfactant   Active surface agent that acts to decrease surface tension, thereby allowing easier ventilation of the alveoli; believed to be secreted by type II alveolar cells.

Sympathetic nervous system   Part of the nervous system that supplies innervation to the visceral and musculoskeletal system. Its primary hormone transmitter is norepinephrine. Sympathetic innervation to the airways facilitates smooth muscle relaxation, thereby causing bronchial dilatation.

Systemic hypertension   Condition in which the patient has a higher-than-normal overall blood pressure.

Systole   Ventricular contraction that ejects blood into the arterial system. The left ventricle ejects into the aorta, and the right ventricle ejects into the pulmonary artery.

Systolic crescendo murmur   Heart sound that begins as a faint sound, then rises in volume; occurs during the ventricular contraction phase of the cardiac cycle.

Systolic ejection murmur   Murmur heard in systole that is caused by turbulent blood flow as the right or left ventricle ejects blood; it can be an innocent murmur.

Systolic regurgitation murmur   Sound created by turbulent backward blood flow from either the mitral or tricuspid valve during the ventricular contraction phase of the cardiac cycle.

T_1   Tricuspid component of S_1.

Terminal respiratory bronchioles   Final part of the conducting airways. They mark the beginning of the respiratory zone.

Thoracic cavity   Space within the rib cage that begins at the clavicle and ends at the diaphragm.

Thorax Bony structure that encloses the thoracic cavity, protecting the heart, lungs, and great vessels.

3LSB Third intercostal space, left sternal border (Erb's point).

Thrill Abnormal tremor felt on palpation that accompanies a vascular or cardiac murmur.

Tilting-disk valve Prosthetic heart valve characterized by a disk that tilts with ventricular pressure to open and close the valvular opening.

TP interval Portion of the ECG tracing between the end of the T wave and the beginning of the P wave.

Tracheal breath sound Loud, tubular (hollow) breath sound auscultated over the trachea that is audible during inspiration and expiration.

Tracheobronchial tree Portion of the airway that begins at the larynx and ends at the terminal bronchioles; also known as the *lower airway*.

Tricuspid insufficiency Tricuspid valve incompetence during systole, which allows turbulent backward, or regurgitant, blood flow into the right atrium.

Tricuspid stenosis Narrowing or constriction of the tricuspid valve.

Tricuspid valve Heart valve between the right atrium and right ventricle.

Tubular breath sound Loud, hollow sound characteristically heard over the trachea and mainstem bronchi.

Turbinate *See* Conchae.

Turbulence Disturbed or irregular airflow; can be caused by rapid flow rates or variations in air pressures and velocities.

2LSB Second intercostal space, left sternal border (pulmonic area).

2RSB Second intercostal space, right sternal border (aortic area).

T wave Part of the ECG tracing that represents ventricular repolarization.

Type I alveolar cell One of three cell types that make up the alveoli; covers approximately 95% of the alveolar surface area.

Type II alveolar cell One of three cell types that line the alveoli; believed to be involved in producing surfactant.

Valsalva's maneuver Attempt to exhale forcibly with the glottis closed.

Ventilation Movement of air in and out of the lungs.

Ventricular ejection Ventricular contraction that sends blood into the arterial system; called systole in the cardiac cycle.

Ventricular filling Ventricular relaxation and expansion that allows blood to enter; called diastole in the cardiac cycle.

Ventricular outflow obstruction Blockage in the valve or vessel that carries blood out of one of the heart's ventricles.

Ventricular septal defect Opening in the septum between the ventricles; usually represents a congenital abnormality.

Ventricular tachycardia Rapid heart rate originating in an ectopic focus in the ventricle.

Vesicular sounds Term frequently used to describe normal breath sounds auscultated over most of the chest wall.

Vocal cord One of two membranous structures in the larynx responsible for phonation.

Vortex Circular airflow caused by the shearing force of high-velocity airstreams alongside slower airstreams. Vortices within the airways are precipitated by airway branching that causes airflow to change direction abruptly.

Wheeze Continuous, high-pitched sound that has a musical quality.

Whispered pectoriloquy High-frequency whispered voice sound auscultated over consolidated or atelectatic areas.

Index

A

Abnormal breath sounds,
34-75. *See also specific
type.*
Absent breath sounds
conditions related to,
45-51
production of, 44
Accessory muscles of respiration, 10
Acetylcholine, lower airway
innervation and, 7
Acoustical mismatch, 240
Acute mitral regurgitation
murmurs, 151-152
auscultatory area for, 151,
151i
characteristics of, 151-152,
152i
Acute pulmonary hypertension, 240
Adrenergic beta$_2$-receptors,
lower airway and, 7-8
Adult respiratory distress
syndrome, 240
Adventitious sounds
classifying, 24, 54-55
crackles as, 56-66
Airflow pattern
during expiration, 3, 4i
during inspiration, 2-3, 3i
in nasal cavity, 3-4, 4i
postural changes and, 12
variations in, 21, 21i
Airway obstruction, absent
breath sounds and, 45i,
46-47, 46i
Alveolar-capillary membrane,
carbon dioxide-oxygen
exchange at, 3, 3i, 4i,
6-7
Alveolar duct, 7i
Alveoli, 6-7, 7i
types of, 6
Anatomic dead space, 5
Anterior axillary line as landmark, 13, 13i

Antigen, 240
Aortic area as auscultatory
site, 84, 85i, 86, 86i
Aortic ball-in-cage valve,
171-172
auscultatory area for, 171
characteristics of, 171-172,
172i
detecting malfunction in,
172
Aortic bileaflet valve,
173-174
auscultatory area for, 173
characteristics of, 173,
173i
detecting malfunction in,
174
Aortic ejections sounds,
130-131
area producing, 128i
auscultatory area for, 130,
130i
characteristics of, 130-131
differentiating, from other
heart sounds, 131
relationship of, to ECG,
131, 131i
Aortic insufficiency. *See* Early diastolic aortic regurgitation mumurs.
Aortic porcine valve, 174
auscultatory area for, 174
characteristics of, 174,
174i
detecting malfunction in,
174
Aortic prosthetic valves,
171-174
abnormal heart sounds in,
182t
auscultatory area for, 171i
malfunctioning
abnormal breath sounds
in, 184t
abnormal heart sounds
in, 184t

i refers to an illustration; t refers to a table.

i refers to an illustration; t refers to a table.

i refers to an illustration; t refers to a table.

i refers to an illustration; t refers to a table.

i refers to an illustration; t refers to a table.

i refers to an illustration; t refers to a table.

i refers to an illustration; t refers to a table.

Tricuspid stenosis, abnormal heart sounds in, 187t
Tricuspid stenosis murmurs, 163-164
  area producing, 163i
  auscultatory area for, 163, 164i
  characteristics of, 163-164, 164i
Turbinates, 3, 4i
Turbulent airflow, pattern of, 21, 21i
T wave, significance of, 97, 97i

U

Upper airway, anatomy of, 3-4, 3i

V

Vagal nerve fibers, lower airway and, 7
Ventilation, distribution of, during breathing, 11, 12
Ventricular filling sounds, 115
Ventricular gallop, 117. *See also* S₃, abnormal.
Ventricular outflow obstruction murmurs, 140-147
Ventricular septal defect, 260
  abnormal heart sounds in, 187t
Ventricular septal defect murmur, 154, 154i
Vertebral column, 9i
Vertebral line as landmark, 13, 14i
Vesicular breath sounds. *See* Normal breath sounds.
Vocal cords, 5i
Voice sounds
  abnormal
    auscultatory sites for, 40, 40i, 41, 41i, 42, 42i
    characteristics of, 40-42
    consolidation and, 42
    production of, 39
    types of, 39-42
  classifying, 24
  damping and, 22
Vortices, pattern of, 21, 21i

WXYZ
Wheezes, 68-75
  conditions associated with, 69
  expiratory polyphonic, 69-70, 70i
  fixed monophonic, 70-71, 71i
  random monophonic, 72-74, 74i, 75i
  sequential inspiratory, 71-72, 72i
  sound production and, 68-69
  stridor and, 74-75
  transmission of, 69
Whispered pectoriloquy, 24, 41
  area producing, 41, 41i
  auscultatory sites for, 41, 41i
  sound characteristics of, 41-42
Whooping cough, abnormal breath sounds in, 187t

i refers to an illustration; t refers to a table.